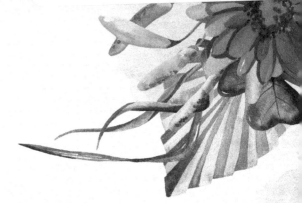

AYURVEDA

THE WISDOM OF LONGEVITY

Design the life you want to live.
Create moments of balance & bliss.
Connect to your true nature.

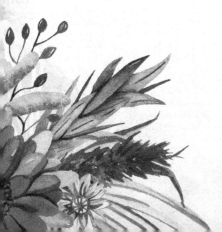

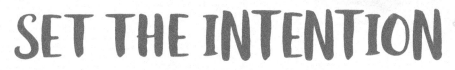

SET THE INTENTION

WHAT ARE YOU WANTING TO CREATE THIS YEAR?

....

....

....

....

....

....

....

....

....

....

....

VALUES/INTENTIONS: *abundance, authenticity, autonomy, balance, beauty, boldness, compassion, community, crea-tivity, curiosity, faith, friendship, growth, happiness, humor, justice, kindness, leadership, learn-ing, love, pleasure, respect, service, spirituality, stability, trust, & wisdom.*

Your Dosha is your mind-body constitution. Particular elements, physical, and emotional characteristics combine to create beautiful, unique, exceptional you! Once you know your Dosha, you'll have a better idea of where you're likely to fall out of balance and what tools to use to return to a harmonious state. You'll be a blend of v. (Vata), p. (Pitta) and k. (Kapha), but most likely one or two will stand out most. Take this quiz to find out what Doshas are most present within you.

1. **FRAME:** V. I HAVE SMALL BONES AND IT'S HARD FOR ME TO GAIN WEIGHT. P. I HAVE MEDIUM BONES, AND I'M FAIRLY MUSCULAR. K. I HAVE BIG BONES AND GAIN WEIGHT EASILY.

2. **SKIN:** V. MY SKIN IS DRY. P. MY SKIN IS OILY; I HAVE FRECKLES, MOLES, OR OCCASIONAL PIMPLES. K. MY SKIN IS THICK AND MOIST.

3. **DIGESTION:** V. MY APPETITE VARIES; I SOMETIMES FORGET TO EAT AND GET GASSY AND BLOATED. P. I HAVE A GOOD APPETITE AND I GET ANGRY WHEN I'M NOT FED. K. I HAVE SLOW DIGESTION; I'M RARELY HUNGRY FOR BREAKFAST.

4. **PERSONALITY:** V. I AM CREATIVE; PEOPLE CALL ME A BUSY BODY. P. I AM AMBITIOUS AND COMPETITIVE K. I AM LAID BACK; PEOPLE SAY I'M A SUPPORT FRIEND; THEY CALL ME THE ROCK OF THE GROUP.

5. **STRESS:** V. I GET ANXIOUS WHEN I'M STRESSED. P. I BECOME IRRITABLE AND DETERMINED UNDER STRESS. K. I'M RARELY STRESSED.

6. **IMBALANCES:** V. I'M PRONE TO ANXIETY, INSOMNIA, AND CONSTIPATION. P. I'M PRONE TO HEARTBURN, ACID REFLUX, SKIN ISSUES, AND IMPATIENCE. K. I'M PRONE TO WATER RETENTION, WEIGHT GAIN, AND COMPLACENCY.

7. **MONEY:** V. I SPEND SPONTANEOUSLY ON WHATEVER CATCHES MY EYE; SOMETIMES I'M LOW ON CASH. B. I SPEND MOSTLY ON LUXURIOUS ITEMS OR ITEMS THAT WILL PROMOTE MY EDUCATIONAL OR CAREER STA-TUS. C. I'M A SAVER; I MANAGE MONEY WELL.

8. **IDEAL VOCATION:** V. I'D LOVE TO BE A WRITER, DANCER, OR MUSICIAN. P. I STRIVE TO BE THE BEST AT WHATEVER I DO—BUSINESS, POLITICS, OR MEDICINE. K. I LOVE TAKING CARE OF PEOPLE; I'D BE A GREAT NURSE, CHEF, OR PARENT OF THE YEAR.

9. **SLEEP:** V. I'M A LIGHT SLEEPER/ PRONE TO INSOMNIA. P. I MIGHT WAKE UP IN THE MIDDLE OF THE NIGHT, BUT I'LL FALL BACK TO SLEEP. I HAVE TO WAKE UP AT A SET TIME BECAUSE I HAVE A LOT TO ACCOMPLISH. K. I AM A SOUND SLEEPER. I LOVE SLEEPING IN.

10. **DECISION MAKING:** V. I MAKE DECISIONS SPONTANEOUSLY, BUT OFTEN CHANGE MY MIND. OTHER TIMES I CANNOT DECIDE. P. I ANALYZE MY CHOICES, AND STICK TO MY DECISIONS. K. I LET OTHER PEOPLE DE-CIDE; I'M GENERALLY CONTENT WITH WHAT PEOPLE CHOOSE.

Each Dosha governs a particular season, depending on where you live Vata season is about October-February, Kapha season is generally March through May, and Pitta Season is June-early September. Learn more as you turn the pages and play around with the concepts.

MY IDEAL
ROUTINE

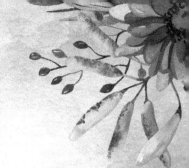

6:00 AM
WAKE UP *sunrise*

6:30 AM
MOVE

7:15 AM
MEDITATE

7:45 AM
BREAKFAST

8:30 AM
WORK

10:30 AM

fill in the blank

12:00 PM
LUNCH

my biggest meal

2:00 PM

fill in the blank

5:00 PM
DINNER

my lightest meal. so grounding

6:30 AM
NIGHTLY ROUTINE

(golden milk)

10:00 PM
SWEET DREAMS

(self massage with oil)

(soothing shower)

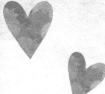

Vata Season

FALL-EARLY WINTER/VATA SEASON/ OCTOBER- FEBRUARY *(ruling elements: ether & air)* *The atmosphere is cool, windy and dry. Vata is up! People are more prone towards: constipation, low back pain, dry/cracking joints, anxiety, insomnia, and insecurity.*

THE REMEDY

- [ ] Stick to a schedule.
- [ ] Slow down.
- [ ] Take time to rest.
- [ ] Walk bare footed on the earth.
- [ ] Take an epsom salt bath.
- [ ] Drink Golden Milk. (turmeric, ginger, nutmeg, cardamom, and cinnamon by wellBlends)
- [ ] Meditate. (Try Insight Timer, guided meditations)
- [ ] Practice Hatha Yoga or take a walk in the forest.
- [ ] Sleep with a weighted blanket or big pillow on your pelvis.
- [ ] Give yourself an oil massage using refined sesame oil before you shower.

NUTRITION

for Vata Season

Eat warm, moist, spiced foods—such as stir-fry, roasted root vegetables, stews, and oatmeal.

Drink hot water with lemon, chamomile and tulsi tea.

Ayurvedic Tea made with ginger, cumin, coriander, and fennel will help mitigate holiday induced digestive discomfort.

....

....

....

....

....

January

TO DO:

- ●
- ●
- ●
- ●
- ●
- ●
- ●
- ●
- ●
- ●
- ●
- ●
- ●

SUNDAY	MONDAY	TUESDAY
☐	☐	☐
3	4 Balance	5
10	11	12
17	18	19
24 Mellow	25	26
31	☐	☐

WEDNESDAY	THURSDAY	FRIDAY	SATURDAY
☐	☐	1	2
6	7 *Ground*	8	9
13	14	15	16
20	21	22	23
27	28	29 *Slow Down*	30
☐	☐	☐	☐

I am grounded.

MONDAY	TUESDAY	WEDNESDAY
December 28	December 29	December 30

MONDAY — December 28

- ☐ ....
- ☐ ....
- ☐ ....
- ☐ ....
- ☐ ....
- ☐ ....
- ☐ ....
- ☐ ....
- ☐ ....
- ☐ ....
- ☐ ....
- ☐ ....
- ☐ ....

TUESDAY — December 29

- ☐ ....
- ☐ ....
- ☐ ....
- ☐ ....
- ☐ ....
- ☐ ....
- ☐ ....
- ☐ ....
- ☐ ....
- ☐ ....
- ☐ ....
- ☐ ....
- ☐ ....
- ☐ ....

WEDNESDAY — December 30

- ☐ ....
- ☐ ....
- ☐ ....
- ☐ ....
- ☐ ....
- ☐ ....
- ☐ ....
- ☐ ....
- ☐ ....
- ☐ ....
- ☐ ....
- ☐ ....
- ☐ ....

Ground with routines & self-care. I commit to _____ in the morning and _____ at night. My Affirmations this week are: _____ _____. I will repeat them when I wake up and before I go to sleep.

THURSDAY	FRIDAY	WEEKEND
December 31	January 1	January 2-3
☐	☐	☐ ....
☐	☐	☐ ....
☐	☐	☐ ....
☐	☐	☐ ....
☐	☐	☐ ....
☐	☐	☐ ....
☐	☐	☐ ....
☐	☐	☐ ....
☐	☐	☐ ....
☐	☐	☐ ....
☐	☐	☐ ....
☐	☐	☐ ....
☐	☐	☐ ....

I am calm.

MONDAY
January 4

- ☐ ....
- ☐ ....
- ☐ ....
- ☐ ....
- ☐ ....
- ☐ ....
- ☐ ....
- ☐ ....
- ☐ ....
- ☐ ....
- ☐ ....
- ☐ ....
- ☐ ....

TUESDAY
January 5

- ☐ ....
- ☐ ....
- ☐ ....
- ☐ ....
- ☐ ....
- ☐ ....
- ☐ ....
- ☐ ....
- ☐ ....
- ☐ ....
- ☐ ....
- ☐ ....
- ☐ ....
- ☐ ....

WEDNESDAY
January 6

- ☐ ....
- ☐ ....
- ☐ ....
- ☐ ....
- ☐ ....
- ☐ ....
- ☐ ....
- ☐ ....
- ☐ ....
- ☐ ....
- ☐ ....
- ☐ ....
- ☐ ....

Ground with routines & self-care. I commit to _____ in the morning and _____ at night. My Affirmations this week are: _____ _____. I will repeat them when I wake up and before I go to sleep.

THURSDAY	FRIDAY	WEEKEND
January 7	January 8	January 9-10

THURSDAY — January 7
- ☐ ....
- ☐ ....
- ☐ ....
- ☐ ....
- ☐ ....
- ☐ ....
- ☐ ....
- ☐ ....
- ☐ ....
- ☐ ....
- ☐ ....
- ☐ ....
- ☐ ....
- ☐ ....

FRIDAY — January 8
- ☐ ....
- ☐ ....
- ☐ ....
- ☐ ....
- ☐ ....
- ☐ ....
- ☐ ....
- ☐ ....
- ☐ ....
- ☐ ....
- ☐ ....
- ☐ ....
- ☐ ....

WEEKEND — January 9-10
- ☐ ....
- ☐ ....
- ☐ ....
- ☐ ....
- ☐ ....
- ☐ ....
- ☐ ....
- ☐ ....
- ☐ ....
- ☐ ....
- ☐ ....
- ☐ ....
- ☐ ....

I am loved.

MONDAY	TUESDAY	WEDNESDAY
January 11	January 12	January 13

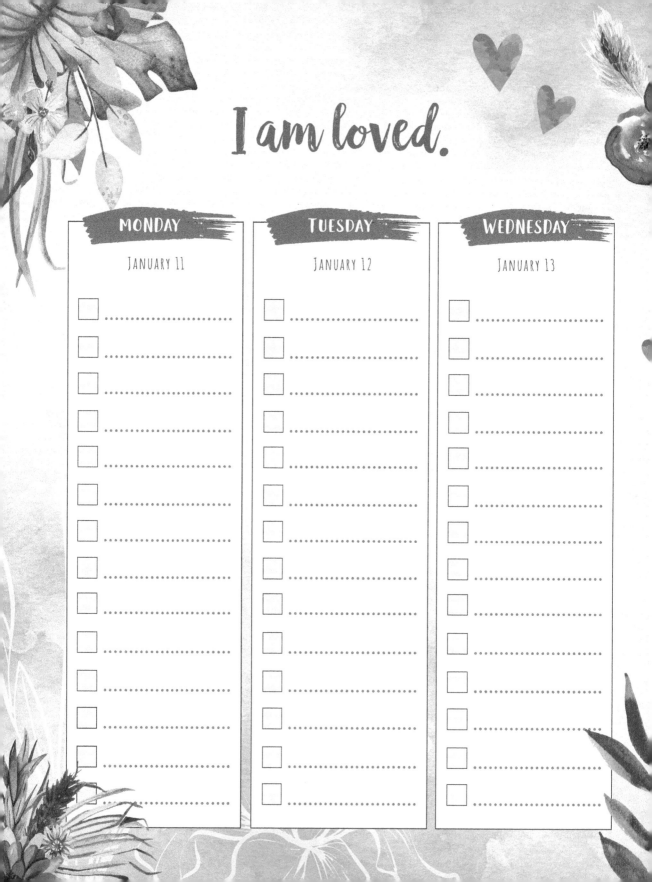

Ground with routines & self-care. I commit to _____ in the morning and _____ at night. My Affirmations this week are: _____ _____. I will repeat them when I wake up and before I go to sleep.

THURSDAY

JANUARY 14

- ☐ ....
- ☐ ....
- ☐ ....
- ☐ ....
- ☐ ....
- ☐ ....
- ☐ ....
- ☐ ....
- ☐ ....
- ☐ ....
- ☐ ....
- ☐ ....
- ☐ ....

FRIDAY

JANUARY 15

- ☐ ....
- ☐ ....
- ☐ ....
- ☐ ....
- ☐ ....
- ☐ ....
- ☐ ....
- ☐ ....
- ☐ ....
- ☐ ....
- ☐ ....
- ☐ ....
- ☐ ....

WEEKEND

JANUARY 16-17

- ☐ ....
- ☐ ....
- ☐ ....
- ☐ ....
- ☐ ....
- ☐ ....
- ☐ ....
- ☐ ....
- ☐ ....
- ☐ ....
- ☐ ....
- ☐ ....

I am whole.

MONDAY	TUESDAY	WEDNESDAY
January 18	January 19	January 20

MONDAY — January 18
- [ ] ....
- [ ] ....
- [ ] ....
- [ ] ....
- [ ] ....
- [ ] ....
- [ ] ....
- [ ] ....
- [ ] ....
- [ ] ....
- [ ] ....
- [ ] ....
- [ ] ....

TUESDAY — January 19
- [ ] ....
- [ ] ....
- [ ] ....
- [ ] ....
- [ ] ....
- [ ] ....
- [ ] ....
- [ ] ....
- [ ] ....
- [ ] ....
- [ ] ....
- [ ] ....
- [ ] ....
- [ ] ....

WEDNESDAY — January 20
- [ ] ....
- [ ] ....
- [ ] ....
- [ ] ....
- [ ] ....
- [ ] ....
- [ ] ....
- [ ] ....
- [ ] ....
- [ ] ....
- [ ] ....
- [ ] ....
- [ ] ....

Ground with routines & self-care. I commit to _____ in the morning and _____ at night. My Affirmations this week are: _____ _____. I will repeat them when I wake up and before I go to sleep.

THURSDAY

JANUARY 21

- [ ] ....
- [ ] ....
- [ ] ....
- [ ] ....
- [ ] ....
- [ ] ....
- [ ] ....
- [ ] ....
- [ ] ....
- [ ] ....
- [ ] ....
- [ ] ....
- [ ] ....

FRIDAY

JANUARY 22

- [ ] ....
- [ ] ....
- [ ] ....
- [ ] ....
- [ ] ....
- [ ] ....
- [ ] ....
- [ ] ....
- [ ] ....
- [ ] ....
- [ ] ....
- [ ] ....
- [ ] ....
- [ ] ....

WEEKEND

JANUARY 23-24

- [ ] ....
- [ ] ....
- [ ] ....
- [ ] ....
- [ ] ....
- [ ] ....
- [ ] ....
- [ ] ....
- [ ] ....
- [ ] ....
- [ ] ....
- [ ] ....
- [ ] ....

I am mindful.

MONDAY	TUESDAY	WEDNESDAY
January 25	January 26	January 27

☐ ....
☐ ....
☐ ....
☐ ....
☐ ....
☐ ....
☐ ....
☐ ....
☐ ....
☐ ....
☐ ....
☐ ....
☐ ....

Ground with routines & self-care. I commit to _____ in the morning and _____ at night. My Affirmations this week are: _____ _____. I will repeat them when I wake up and before I go to sleep.

THURSDAY	FRIDAY	WEEKEND
January 28	January 29	January 30-31

☐ ....
☐ ....
☐ ....
☐ ....
☐ ....
☐ ....
☐ ....
☐ ....
☐ ....
☐ ....
☐ ....
☐ ....
☐ ....

ROASTED ROOT VEGETABLES WITH THYME

INGREDIENTS

- Nonstick coconut oil spray
- 1 pound red-skinned potatoes, unpeeled, scrubbed, cut into 1-inch pieces
- 1 pound celery root (celeriac), peeled, cut into 1-inch pieces
- 1 pound rutabagas, peeled, cut into 1-inch pieces
- 1 pound carrots, peeled, cut into 1-inch pieces
- 1 pound parsnips, peeled, cut into 1-inch pieces
- 2 onions, cut into 1-inch pieces
- 2 leeks (white and pale green parts only), cut into 1-inch-thick rounds
- 2 tablespoons chopped fresh rosemary
- 1/2 cup olive oil
- 10 garlic cloves, peeled

DIRECTIONS

Position 1 rack in bottom third of oven and 1 rack in center of oven and preheat to 400°F. Spray 2 heavy large baking sheets with nonstick spray. Combine all remaining ingredients except garlic in very large bowl; toss to coat. Season generously with salt and pepper. Divide vegetable mixture between prepared sheets. Place 1 sheet on each oven rack. Roast 30 minutes, stirring occasionally. Reverse positions of baking sheets. Add 5 garlic cloves to each baking sheet. Continue to roast until all vegetables are tender and brown in spots, stirring and turning vegetables occasionally, about 45 minutes longer. (Can be prepared 4 hours ahead. Let stand on baking sheets at room temperature. Rewarm in 450°F oven until heated through, about 15 minutes.) Transfer roasted vegetables to large bowl and then serve.

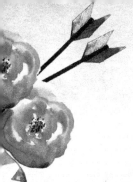

SQUASH CURRY

INGREDIENTS

- 1½ cups butternut squash, yams, or sweet potatoes

- 1 tablespoon raisins (soaked in water for 15 minutes)

- 2 teaspoons crushed cashews

- 1 teaspoon brown sugar

- 1 tablespoon minced cilantro leaves

- ½ teaspoon salt

- 1 tablespoon ghee

- 2 teaspoons curry spices

DIRECTIONS

Bake or steam squash. Sauté curry spices in ghee. Add cashews, brown sugar, and raisins. Cube or mash squash and add to mixture. Add salt and cilantro. Cook for 5 minutes. Serve with rice

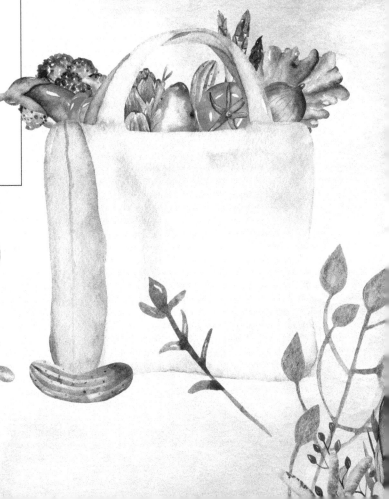

MEAL PREP:

- SWEET POTATOES
- SQUASH
- CARROTS
- DATES
- OATMEAL
- APPLES
- CINNAMON
- GOLDEN MILK
- SPINACH
- BROWN RICE
- CHICKEN BROTH

I'M MAKING:

- SWEET POTATOE CHILI
- ROASTED ROOT VEGETABLES
- OATMEAL WITH CINNAMON AND DATES
- ☐ ....
- ☐ ....
- ☐ ....
- ☐ ....
- ☐ ....

VATA STRENGHTS

Creative
....
Adaptable
....
Energetic
....
Excitable
....
Intuitive
....

MY STRENGTHS RIGHT NOW:

Journal

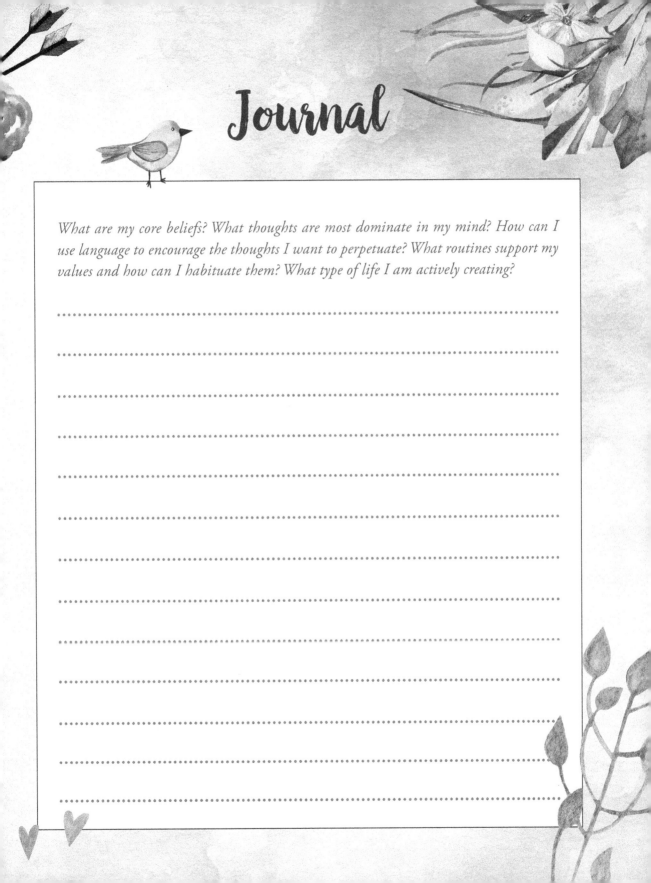

What are my core beliefs? What thoughts are most dominate in my mind? How can I use language to encourage the thoughts I want to perpetuate? What routines support my values and how can I habituate them? What type of life I am actively creating?

....

....

....

....

....

....

....

....

....

....

....

....

"Your beliefs become your thoughts. Your thoughts become your words, Your words become your actions, your actions become your habits, your habits become your values, your values become your destiny."

—MAHATMA GANDHI

February

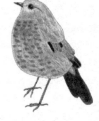

TO DO:

-
-
-
-
-
-
-
-
-
-
-
-
-

SUNDAY	MONDAY	TUESDAY
	1	2
7 Breathe	8	9
14	15	16 Feel
21	22	23
28		

WEDNESDAY	THURSDAY	FRIDAY	SATURDAY
3	4	5	6
10	11 *Relax*	12	13
17	18	19	20
24	25	26 *Love*	27
☐	☐	☐	☐

I am taking care of myself today.

MONDAY	TUESDAY	WEDNESDAY
February 1	February 2	February 3

MONDAY — February 1
- ☐ ....
- ☐ ....
- ☐ ....
- ☐ ....
- ☐ ....
- ☐ ....
- ☐ ....
- ☐ ....
- ☐ ....
- ☐ ....
- ☐ ....
- ☐ ....
- ☐ ....

TUESDAY — February 2
- ☐ ....
- ☐ ....
- ☐ ....
- ☐ ....
- ☐ ....
- ☐ ....
- ☐ ....
- ☐ ....
- ☐ ....
- ☐ ....
- ☐ ....
- ☐ ....
- ☐ ....
- ☐ ....

WEDNESDAY — February 3
- ☐ ....
- ☐ ....
- ☐ ....
- ☐ ....
- ☐ ....
- ☐ ....
- ☐ ....
- ☐ ....
- ☐ ....
- ☐ ....
- ☐ ....
- ☐ ....
- ☐ ....

Ground with routines & self-care. I commit to _____ in the morning and _____ at night. My Affirmations this week are: _____ _____. I will repeat them when I wake up and before I go to sleep.

THURSDAY

February 4

- [ ] ....
- [ ] ....
- [ ] ....
- [ ] ....
- [ ] ....
- [ ] ....
- [ ] ....
- [ ] ....
- [ ] ....
- [ ] ....
- [ ] ....
- [ ] ....
- [ ] ....

FRIDAY

February 5

- [ ] ....
- [ ] ....
- [ ] ....
- [ ] ....
- [ ] ....
- [ ] ....
- [ ] ....
- [ ] ....
- [ ] ....
- [ ] ....
- [ ] ....
- [ ] ....
- [ ] ....

WEEKEND

February 6-7

- [ ] ....
- [ ] ....
- [ ] ....
- [ ] ....
- [ ] ....
- [ ] ....
- [ ] ....
- [ ] ....
- [ ] ....
- [ ] ....
- [ ] ....
- [ ] ....
- [ ] ....

I am connected to the earth.

MONDAY	TUESDAY	WEDNESDAY
February 8	February 9	February 10

MONDAY — February 8

- ☐ ....
- ☐ ....
- ☐ ....
- ☐ ....
- ☐ ....
- ☐ ....
- ☐ ....
- ☐ ....
- ☐ ....
- ☐ ....
- ☐ ....
- ☐ ....
- ☐ ....
- ☐ ....

TUESDAY — February 9

- ☐ ....
- ☐ ....
- ☐ ....
- ☐ ....
- ☐ ....
- ☐ ....
- ☐ ....
- ☐ ....
- ☐ ....
- ☐ ....
- ☐ ....
- ☐ ....
- ☐ ....
- ☐ ....

WEDNESDAY — February 10

- ☐ ....
- ☐ ....
- ☐ ....
- ☐ ....
- ☐ ....
- ☐ ....
- ☐ ....
- ☐ ....
- ☐ ....
- ☐ ....
- ☐ ....
- ☐ ....
- ☐ ....
- ☐ ....

Ground with routines & self-care. I commit to _____ in the morning and _____ at night. My Affirmations this week are: _____
_____. I will repeat them when I wake up and before I go to sleep.

THURSDAY	FRIDAY	WEEKEND
February 11	February 12	February 13-14

THURSDAY — February 11

- ☐ ....
- ☐ ....
- ☐ ....
- ☐ ....
- ☐ ....
- ☐ ....
- ☐ ....
- ☐ ....
- ☐ ....
- ☐ ....
- ☐ ....
- ☐ ....
- ☐ ....
- ☐ ....

FRIDAY — February 12

- ☐ ....
- ☐ ....
- ☐ ....
- ☐ ....
- ☐ ....
- ☐ ....
- ☐ ....
- ☐ ....
- ☐ ....
- ☐ ....
- ☐ ....
- ☐ ....
- ☐ ....

WEEKEND — February 13-14

- ☐ ....
- ☐ ....
- ☐ ....
- ☐ ....
- ☐ ....
- ☐ ....
- ☐ ....
- ☐ ....
- ☐ ....
- ☐ ....
- ☐ ....
- ☐ ....
- ☐ ....

I am spending time in nature.

MONDAY	TUESDAY	WEDNESDAY
February 15	February 16	February 17
☐	☐	☐ ....
☐	☐	☐ ....
☐	☐	☐ ....
☐	☐	☐ ....
☐	☐	☐ ....
☐	☐	☐ ....
☐	☐	☐ ....
☐	☐	☐ ....
☐	☐	☐ ....
☐	☐	☐ ....
☐	☐	☐ ....
☐	☐	☐ ....
☐	☐	☐ ....

Ground with routines & self-care. I commit to _____ in the morning and _____ at night. My Affirmations this week are: _____ _____. I will repeat them when I wake up and before I go to sleep.

THURSDAY

February 18

- ☐ ....
- ☐ ....
- ☐ ....
- ☐ ....
- ☐ ....
- ☐ ....
- ☐ ....
- ☐ ....
- ☐ ....
- ☐ ....
- ☐ ....
- ☐ ....
- ☐ ....

FRIDAY

February 19

- ☐ ....
- ☐ ....
- ☐ ....
- ☐ ....
- ☐ ....
- ☐ ....
- ☐ ....
- ☐ ....
- ☐ ....
- ☐ ....
- ☐ ....
- ☐ ....
- ☐ ....

WEEKEND

February 20-21

- ☐ ....
- ☐ ....
- ☐ ....
- ☐ ....
- ☐ ....
- ☐ ....
- ☐ ....
- ☐ ....
- ☐ ....
- ☐ ....
- ☐ ....
- ☐ ....
- ☐ ....

I am at peace.

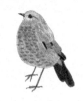

MONDAY	TUESDAY	WEDNESDAY
February 22	February 23	February 24

MONDAY — February 22

- ☐ ....
- ☐ ....
- ☐ ....
- ☐ ....
- ☐ ....
- ☐ ....
- ☐ ....
- ☐ ....
- ☐ ....
- ☐ ....
- ☐ ....
- ☐ ....
- ☐ ....

TUESDAY — February 23

- ☐ ....
- ☐ ....
- ☐ ....
- ☐ ....
- ☐ ....
- ☐ ....
- ☐ ....
- ☐ ....
- ☐ ....
- ☐ ....
- ☐ ....
- ☐ ....
- ☐ ....

WEDNESDAY — February 24

- ☐ ....
- ☐ ....
- ☐ ....
- ☐ ....
- ☐ ....
- ☐ ....
- ☐ ....
- ☐ ....
- ☐ ....
- ☐ ....
- ☐ ....
- ☐ ....
- ☐ ....

Ground with routines & self-care. I commit to _____ in the morning and _____ at night. My Affirmations this week are: _____ _____. I will repeat them when I wake up and before I go to sleep.

THURSDAY	FRIDAY	WEEKEND
February 25	February 26	February 27-28

THURSDAY — February 25
- ☐ ....
- ☐ ....
- ☐ ....
- ☐ ....
- ☐ ....
- ☐ ....
- ☐ ....
- ☐ ....
- ☐ ....
- ☐ ....
- ☐ ....
- ☐ ....
- ☐ ....
- ☐ ....

FRIDAY — February 26
- ☐ ....
- ☐ ....
- ☐ ....
- ☐ ....
- ☐ ....
- ☐ ....
- ☐ ....
- ☐ ....
- ☐ ....
- ☐ ....
- ☐ ....
- ☐ ....
- ☐ ....

WEEKEND — February 27-28
- ☐ ....
- ☐ ....
- ☐ ....
- ☐ ....
- ☐ ....
- ☐ ....
- ☐ ....
- ☐ ....
- ☐ ....
- ☐ ....
- ☐ ....
- ☐ ....

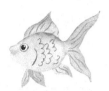

Kapha Season

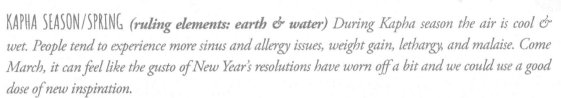

KAPHA SEASON/SPRING *(ruling elements: **earth & water**) During Kapha season the air is cool & wet. People tend to experience more sinus and allergy issues, weight gain, lethargy, and malaise. Come March, it can feel like the gusto of New Year's resolutions have worn off a bit and we could use a good dose of new inspiration.*

THE REMEDY

- [ ] Kick up the digestive flame by drinking ginger tea.

- [ ] Burn away mucus and phlegm by cooking with black pepper, a dash of cayenne, and cinnamon

- [ ] A drizzle of acid (vinegar or lemon).

- [ ] Use invigorating essential oils such as eucalyptus, lemon, and camphor.

- [ ] Get the lymphatic system moving by dry brushing towards the heart. Use a luffa and make quick brush strokes on the body before showering.

- [ ] Move! Find a movement buddy and plan your activity regimens.

- [ ] Cheer each other on. Stay motivated by assigning people to support you.

- [ ] Use "nasya" oil in your nostril am and pm (nasya oil a blend of herbs and sesame oil designed to mitigate allergies).

NUTRITION

for Kapha Season

Avoid heavy and mucus forming foods such as red meat, dairy, sugar, and processed grains like bread and pasta. Eat tons of cooked leafy greens, steamed veggies, beans, and berries. Cook with heating spices like ginger, cinnamon, and black pepper. Favor warm foods such as broth-based soups and steamed veggies. Aim for 50-60% of each meal to be veggie based. Drink net-tle tea to alleviate water retention and allergies.

....

....

....

....

....

....

March

TO DO:

-
-
-
-
-
-
-
-
-
-
-
-
-

SUNDAY	MONDAY	TUESDAY
	1	2
7	8	9 *Energized*
14	15	16
21 *Light*	22	23
28	29	30

WEDNESDAY	THURSDAY	FRIDAY	SATURDAY
3 Happy	4	5	6
10	11	12	13
17	18	19	20
24	25	26 Detox	27
31	☐	☐	☐

I am inspired.

MONDAY	TUESDAY	WEDNESDAY
March 1	March 2	March 3

My movement schedule this week: Monday _____ Tuesday _____
Wednesday _____ Thursday _____ Friday _____
Sat/Sunday _____
The healthy meal I'm most excited about this week is: _____.

THURSDAY
March 4

- [ ] ....
- [ ] ....
- [ ] ....
- [ ] ....
- [ ] ....
- [ ] ....
- [ ] ....
- [ ] ....
- [ ] ....
- [ ] ....
- [ ] ....
- [ ] ....
- [ ] ....

FRIDAY
March 5

- [ ] ....
- [ ] ....
- [ ] ....
- [ ] ....
- [ ] ....
- [ ] ....
- [ ] ....
- [ ] ....
- [ ] ....
- [ ] ....
- [ ] ....
- [ ] ....
- [ ] ....

WEEKEND
March 6-7

- [ ] ....
- [ ] ....
- [ ] ....
- [ ] ....
- [ ] ....
- [ ] ....
- [ ] ....
- [ ] ....
- [ ] ....
- [ ] ....
- [ ] ....
- [ ] ....
- [ ] ....

I am detoxifying.

MONDAY
March 8

- [ ] ....
- [ ] ....
- [ ] ....
- [ ] ....
- [ ] ....
- [ ] ....
- [ ] ....
- [ ] ....
- [ ] ....
- [ ] ....
- [ ] ....
- [ ] ....
- [ ] ....
- [ ] ....

TUESDAY
March 9

- [ ] ....
- [ ] ....
- [ ] ....
- [ ] ....
- [ ] ....
- [ ] ....
- [ ] ....
- [ ] ....
- [ ] ....
- [ ] ....
- [ ] ....
- [ ] ....
- [ ] ....
- [ ] ....

WEDNESDAY
March 10

- [ ] ....
- [ ] ....
- [ ] ....
- [ ] ....
- [ ] ....
- [ ] ....
- [ ] ....
- [ ] ....
- [ ] ....
- [ ] ....
- [ ] ....
- [ ] ....
- [ ] ....
- [ ] ....

My movement schedule this week: Monday _____ Tuesday _____
Wednesday _____ Thursday _____ Friday _____
Sat/Sunday _____
The healthy meal I'm most excited about this week is: _____.

THURSDAY

March 11

- ☐ ....
- ☐ ....
- ☐ ....
- ☐ ....
- ☐ ....
- ☐ ....
- ☐ ....
- ☐ ....
- ☐ ....
- ☐ ....
- ☐ ....
- ☐ ....
- ☐ ....

FRIDAY

March 12

- ☐ ....
- ☐ ....
- ☐ ....
- ☐ ....
- ☐ ....
- ☐ ....
- ☐ ....
- ☐ ....
- ☐ ....
- ☐ ....
- ☐ ....
- ☐ ....
- ☐ ....

WEEKEND

March 13-14

- ☐ ....
- ☐ ....
- ☐ ....
- ☐ ....
- ☐ ....
- ☐ ....
- ☐ ....
- ☐ ....
- ☐ ....
- ☐ ....
- ☐ ....
- ☐ ....
- ☐ ....

I am light.

MONDAY	TUESDAY	WEDNESDAY
March 15	March 16	March 17

MONDAY — March 15

- ☐ ....
- ☐ ....
- ☐ ....
- ☐ ....
- ☐ ....
- ☐ ....
- ☐ ....
- ☐ ....
- ☐ ....
- ☐ ....
- ☐ ....
- ☐ ....
- ☐ ....

TUESDAY — March 16

- ☐ ....
- ☐ ....
- ☐ ....
- ☐ ....
- ☐ ....
- ☐ ....
- ☐ ....
- ☐ ....
- ☐ ....
- ☐ ....
- ☐ ....
- ☐ ....
- ☐ ....

WEDNESDAY — March 17

- ☐ ....
- ☐ ....
- ☐ ....
- ☐ ....
- ☐ ....
- ☐ ....
- ☐ ....
- ☐ ....
- ☐ ....
- ☐ ....
- ☐ ....
- ☐ ....
- ☐ ....

My movement schedule this week: Monday _____ Tuesday _____
Wednesday _____ Thursday _____ Friday _____
Sat/Sunday _____
The healthy meal I'm most excited about this week is: _____.

THURSDAY

MARCH 18

- ☐ ....
- ☐ ....
- ☐ ....
- ☐ ....
- ☐ ....
- ☐ ....
- ☐ ....
- ☐ ....
- ☐ ....
- ☐ ....
- ☐ ....
- ☐ ....
- ☐ ....

FRIDAY

MARCH 19

- ☐ ....
- ☐ ....
- ☐ ....
- ☐ ....
- ☐ ....
- ☐ ....
- ☐ ....
- ☐ ....
- ☐ ....
- ☐ ....
- ☐ ....
- ☐ ....
- ☐ ....

WEEKEND

MARCH 20-21

- ☐ ....
- ☐ ....
- ☐ ....
- ☐ ....
- ☐ ....
- ☐ ....
- ☐ ....
- ☐ ....
- ☐ ....
- ☐ ....
- ☐ ....
- ☐ ....

I am empowered.

MONDAY	TUESDAY	WEDNESDAY
MARCH 22	MARCH 23	MARCH 24

MONDAY — March 22
- ☐ ....
- ☐ ....
- ☐ ....
- ☐ ....
- ☐ ....
- ☐ ....
- ☐ ....
- ☐ ....
- ☐ ....
- ☐ ....
- ☐ ....
- ☐ ....
- ☐ ....

TUESDAY — March 23
- ☐ ....
- ☐ ....
- ☐ ....
- ☐ ....
- ☐ ....
- ☐ ....
- ☐ ....
- ☐ ....
- ☐ ....
- ☐ ....
- ☐ ....
- ☐ ....
- ☐ ....

WEDNESDAY — March 24
- ☐ ....
- ☐ ....
- ☐ ....
- ☐ ....
- ☐ ....
- ☐ ....
- ☐ ....
- ☐ ....
- ☐ ....
- ☐ ....
- ☐ ....
- ☐ ....
- ☐ ....

My movement schedule this week: Monday _____ Tuesday _____
Wednesday _____ Thursday _____ Friday _____
Sat/Sunday _____
The healthy meal I'm most excited about this week is: _____.

THURSDAY

MARCH 25

☐ ....
☐ ....
☐ ....
☐ ....
☐ ....
☐ ....
☐ ....
☐ ....
☐ ....
☐ ....
☐ ....
☐ ....
☐ ....

FRIDAY

MARCH 26

☐ ....
☐ ....
☐ ....
☐ ....
☐ ....
☐ ....
☐ ....
☐ ....
☐ ....
☐ ....
☐ ....
☐ ....
☐ ....

WEEKEND

MARCH 27-28

☐ ....
☐ ....
☐ ....
☐ ....
☐ ....
☐ ....
☐ ....
☐ ....
☐ ....
☐ ....
☐ ....
☐ ....
☐ ....

I am aware.

MONDAY	TUESDAY	WEDNESDAY
March 29	March 30	March 31

MONDAY — March 29

- [ ] ....
- [ ] ....
- [ ] ....
- [ ] ....
- [ ] ....
- [ ] ....
- [ ] ....
- [ ] ....
- [ ] ....
- [ ] ....
- [ ] ....
- [ ] ....
- [ ] ....
- [ ] ....

TUESDAY — March 30

- [ ] ....
- [ ] ....
- [ ] ....
- [ ] ....
- [ ] ....
- [ ] ....
- [ ] ....
- [ ] ....
- [ ] ....
- [ ] ....
- [ ] ....
- [ ] ....
- [ ] ....

WEDNESDAY — March 31

- [ ] ....
- [ ] ....
- [ ] ....
- [ ] ....
- [ ] ....
- [ ] ....
- [ ] ....
- [ ] ....
- [ ] ....
- [ ] ....
- [ ] ....
- [ ] ....
- [ ] ....

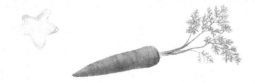

TURMERIC & LENTIL SOUP

INGREDIENTS

- 4 whole CARROT
- 1/2 tsp FENNEL SEEDS
- 1 inch GINGER (FRESH)
- 1/2 lbs KALE
- 1/4 whole LIME
- 1/2 tsp SALT (MINERAL SALT)
- 1 tbsp SUNFLOWER OIL

DIRECTIONS

Chop kale & carrots. Place in a pot and add water until vegetables are just covered. Boil with all ingredients until kale is soft and easy to chew. Easy to chew means easy to digest.

KALE AND CARROT SOUP
with Fennel and Lime

INGREDIENTS

- 1 THINLY SLICED GARLIC CLOVE
- 1.5 TEASPOONS GOLDEN MILK POWDER
- 1/4 TEASPOON TURMERIC AND 1 TEASPOON GRATED GINGER
- 1 TEASPOON EXTRA-VIRGIN OLIVE OIL
- 6 cups Basic Chicken Stock or store-bought low-sodium chicken broth • 3 ounces lentil pasta, broken in half
- 1 cup shredded cooked chicken (optional)
- tablespoon fresh lemon juice
- Microgreens and thinly sliced scallions, for serving

DIRECTIONS

In a saucepan over medium-high heat, sauté garlic, turmeric, and ginger in oil until fragrant, about 30 seconds. Add stock; bring to a simmer. Add pasta; cook 1 minute less than per package in-structions. Add chicken (if using); heat through, 1 minute. Remove from heat. Stir in lemon juice. Serve with micro-greens and scallions

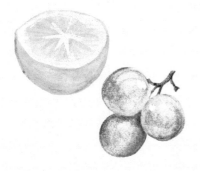

April

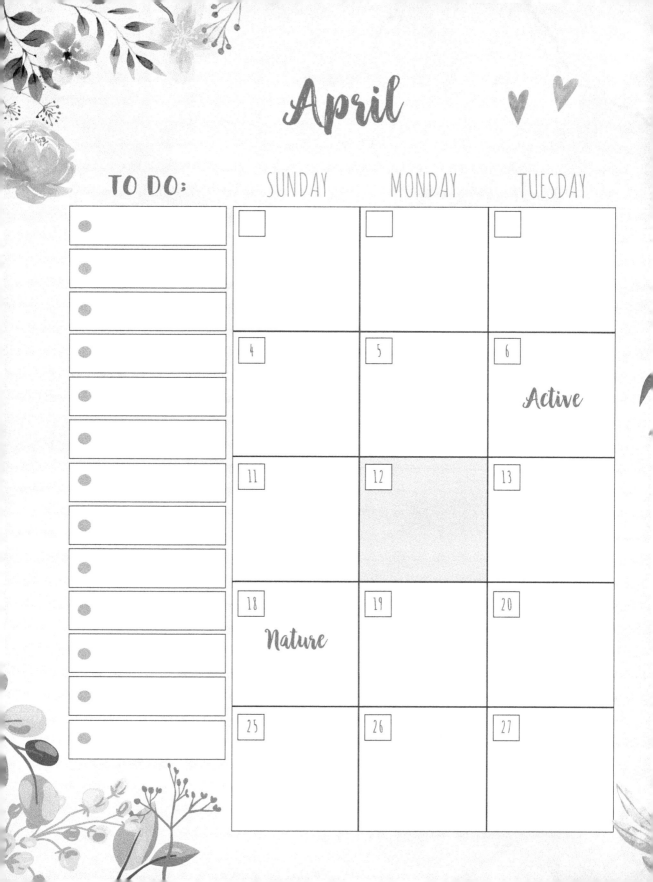

TO DO:

-
-
-
-
-
-
-
-
-
-
-
-
-

SUNDAY	MONDAY	TUESDAY
☐	☐	☐
4	5	6 Active
11	12	13
18 Nature	19	20
25	26	27

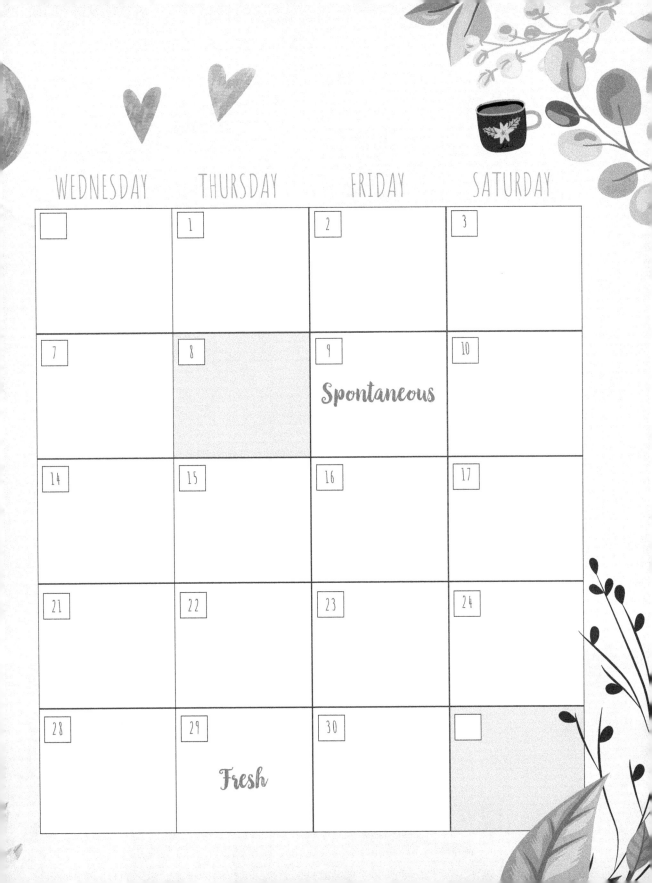

WEDNESDAY	THURSDAY	FRIDAY	SATURDAY
	1	2	3
7	8	9 Spontaneous	10
14	15	16	17
21	22	23	24
28	29 Fresh	30	

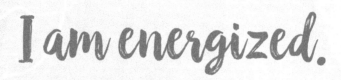 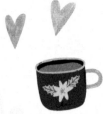

I am energized.

MONDAY	TUESDAY	WEDNESDAY
March 29	March 30	March 31
☐	☐	☐ ....
☐	☐	☐ ....
☐	☐	☐ ....
☐	☐	☐ ....
☐	☐	☐ ....
☐	☐	☐ ....
☐	☐	☐ ....
☐	☐	☐ ....
☐	☐	☐ ....
☐	☐	☐ ....
☐	☐	☐ ....
☐	☐	☐ ....
☐	☐	☐ ....

My movement schedule this week: Monday _____ Tuesday _____
Wednesday _____ Thursday _____ Friday _____
Sat/Sunday _____
The healthy meal I'm most excited about this week is: _____.

THURSDAY

April 1

- ☐ ....
- ☐ ....
- ☐ ....
- ☐ ....
- ☐ ....
- ☐ ....
- ☐ ....
- ☐ ....
- ☐ ....
- ☐ ....
- ☐ ....
- ☐ ....
- ☐ ....
- ☐ ....

FRIDAY

April 2

- ☐ ....
- ☐ ....
- ☐ ....
- ☐ ....
- ☐ ....
- ☐ ....
- ☐ ....
- ☐ ....
- ☐ ....
- ☐ ....
- ☐ ....
- ☐ ....
- ☐ ....
- ☐ ....

WEEKEND

April 3-4

- ☐ ....
- ☐ ....
- ☐ ....
- ☐ ....
- ☐ ....
- ☐ ....
- ☐ ....
- ☐ ....
- ☐ ....
- ☐ ....
- ☐ ....
- ☐ ....
- ☐ ....

I am happy.

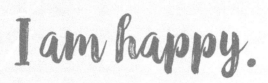
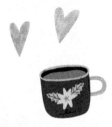

MONDAY	TUESDAY	WEDNESDAY
April 5	April 6	April 7

My movement schedule this week: Monday _____ Tuesday _____
Wednesday _____ Thursday _____ Friday _____
Sat/Sunday _____
The healthy meal I'm most excited about this week is: _____.

THURSDAY

APRIL 8

- [ ] ....
- [ ] ....
- [ ] ....
- [ ] ....
- [ ] ....
- [ ] ....
- [ ] ....
- [ ] ....
- [ ] ....
- [ ] ....
- [ ] ....
- [ ] ....
- [ ] ....
- [ ] ....

FRIDAY

APRIL 9

- [ ] ....
- [ ] ....
- [ ] ....
- [ ] ....
- [ ] ....
- [ ] ....
- [ ] ....
- [ ] ....
- [ ] ....
- [ ] ....
- [ ] ....
- [ ] ....
- [ ] ....
- [ ] ....

WEEKEND

APRIL 10-11

- [ ] ....
- [ ] ....
- [ ] ....
- [ ] ....
- [ ] ....
- [ ] ....
- [ ] ....
- [ ] ....
- [ ] ....
- [ ] ....
- [ ] ....
- [ ] ....
- [ ] ....

I am radiant.

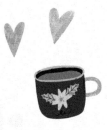

MONDAY
APRIL 12

☐ ....
☐ ....
☐ ....
☐ ....
☐ ....
☐ ....
☐ ....
☐ ....
☐ ....
☐ ....
☐ ....
☐ ....
☐ ....

TUESDAY
APRIL 13

☐ ....
☐ ....
☐ ....
☐ ....
☐ ....
☐ ....
☐ ....
☐ ....
☐ ....
☐ ....
☐ ....
☐ ....
☐ ....

WEDNESDAY
APRIL 14

☐ ....
☐ ....
☐ ....
☐ ....
☐ ....
☐ ....
☐ ....
☐ ....
☐ ....
☐ ....
☐ ....
☐ ....
☐ ....

THURSDAY

APRIL 15

- ☐ ....
- ☐ ....
- ☐ ....
- ☐ ....
- ☐ ....
- ☐ ....
- ☐ ....
- ☐ ....
- ☐ ....
- ☐ ....
- ☐ ....
- ☐ ....
- ☐ ....
- ☐ ....

FRIDAY

APRIL 16

- ☐ ....
- ☐ ....
- ☐ ....
- ☐ ....
- ☐ ....
- ☐ ....
- ☐ ....
- ☐ ....
- ☐ ....
- ☐ ....
- ☐ ....
- ☐ ....
- ☐ ....
- ☐ ....

WEEKEND

APRIL 17-18

- ☐ ....
- ☐ ....
- ☐ ....
- ☐ ....
- ☐ ....
- ☐ ....
- ☐ ....
- ☐ ....
- ☐ ....
- ☐ ....
- ☐ ....
- ☐ ....
- ☐ ....

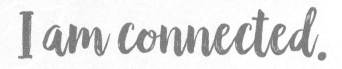 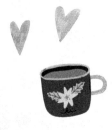

I am connected.

MONDAY	TUESDAY	WEDNESDAY
April 19	April 20	April 21

MONDAY — April 19
- ☐ ....
- ☐ ....
- ☐ ....
- ☐ ....
- ☐ ....
- ☐ ....
- ☐ ....
- ☐ ....
- ☐ ....
- ☐ ....
- ☐ ....
- ☐ ....
- ☐ ....

TUESDAY — April 20
- ☐ ....
- ☐ ....
- ☐ ....
- ☐ ....
- ☐ ....
- ☐ ....
- ☐ ....
- ☐ ....
- ☐ ....
- ☐ ....
- ☐ ....
- ☐ ....
- ☐ ....

WEDNESDAY — April 21
- ☐ ....
- ☐ ....
- ☐ ....
- ☐ ....
- ☐ ....
- ☐ ....
- ☐ ....
- ☐ ....
- ☐ ....
- ☐ ....
- ☐ ....
- ☐ ....
- ☐ ....

My movement schedule this week: Monday _____ Tuesday _____
Wednesday _____ Thursday _____ Friday _____
Sat/Sunday _____
The healthy meal I'm most excited about this week is: _____.

THURSDAY
APRIL 22

- ☐ ....
- ☐ ....
- ☐ ....
- ☐ ....
- ☐ ....
- ☐ ....
- ☐ ....
- ☐ ....
- ☐ ....
- ☐ ....
- ☐ ....
- ☐ ....
- ☐ ....
- ☐ ....

FRIDAY
APRIL 23

- ☐ ....
- ☐ ....
- ☐ ....
- ☐ ....
- ☐ ....
- ☐ ....
- ☐ ....
- ☐ ....
- ☐ ....
- ☐ ....
- ☐ ....
- ☐ ....
- ☐ ....
- ☐ ....

WEEKEND
APRIL 24-25

- ☐ ....
- ☐ ....
- ☐ ....
- ☐ ....
- ☐ ....
- ☐ ....
- ☐ ....
- ☐ ....
- ☐ ....
- ☐ ....
- ☐ ....
- ☐ ....
- ☐ ....
- ☐ ....

I am connected.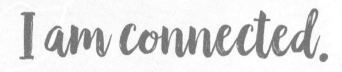

MONDAY	TUESDAY	WEDNESDAY
APRIL 26	APRIL 27	APRIL 28

MONDAY — APRIL 26
- ☐ ....
- ☐ ....
- ☐ ....
- ☐ ....
- ☐ ....
- ☐ ....
- ☐ ....
- ☐ ....
- ☐ ....
- ☐ ....
- ☐ ....
- ☐ ....
- ☐ ....
- ☐ ....

TUESDAY — APRIL 27
- ☐ ....
- ☐ ....
- ☐ ....
- ☐ ....
- ☐ ....
- ☐ ....
- ☐ ....
- ☐ ....
- ☐ ....
- ☐ ....
- ☐ ....
- ☐ ....
- ☐ ....

WEDNESDAY — APRIL 28
- ☐ ....
- ☐ ....
- ☐ ....
- ☐ ....
- ☐ ....
- ☐ ....
- ☐ ....
- ☐ ....
- ☐ ....
- ☐ ....
- ☐ ....
- ☐ ....
- ☐ ....

My movement schedule this week: Monday _____ Tuesday _____
Wednesday _____ Thursday _____ Friday _____
Sat/Sunday _____
The healthy meal I'm most excited about this week is: _____.

THURSDAY

APRIL 29

- [ ] ....
- [ ] ....
- [ ] ....
- [ ] ....
- [ ] ....
- [ ] ....
- [ ] ....
- [ ] ....
- [ ] ....
- [ ] ....
- [ ] ....
- [ ] ....
- [ ] ....
- [ ] ....

FRIDAY

APRIL 30

- [ ] ....
- [ ] ....
- [ ] ....
- [ ] ....
- [ ] ....
- [ ] ....
- [ ] ....
- [ ] ....
- [ ] ....
- [ ] ....
- [ ] ....
- [ ] ....
- [ ] ....
- [ ] ....

WEEKEND

MAY 1-2

- [ ] ....
- [ ] ....
- [ ] ....
- [ ] ....
- [ ] ....
- [ ] ....
- [ ] ....
- [ ] ....
- [ ] ....
- [ ] ....
- [ ] ....
- [ ] ....
- [ ] ....
- [ ] ....

KAPHA STRENGHTS

MEAL PREP:

Loyal

Nurturing

Supportive

Strong

Endurance

MY STRENGTHS RIGHT NOW:

- Kale
- Arugula
- Lentils
- Chickpeas
- Blueberries
- Vegetable Broth
- Quinoa
- Grouper
- Egg Whites
- Lemons
- Black Pepper

I'M MAKING:

- Chickpea Curry
- Lentil Soup
- Steamed Veggies with Fish
- Egg White Omelette with Kale and Peppers
- ☐ ....
- ☐ ....
- ☐ ....
- ☐ ....
- ☐ ....

Meditation

BREATHING & MEDITATION

Breathing through the nose—Inhale breath into the belly and pause. Inhale, continue breath up into chest. Pause. Now both lungs are full. Exhale all the breath. Repeat this 3x.

WALKING MEDITATION

As you enjoy a walk, repeat your affirmations over and over again. If the mind wanders away, bring it back to the repetition of the affirmations as you stroll. For example: "I am loved. I am worthy. I am enough. I am energized. I am enjoying my life."

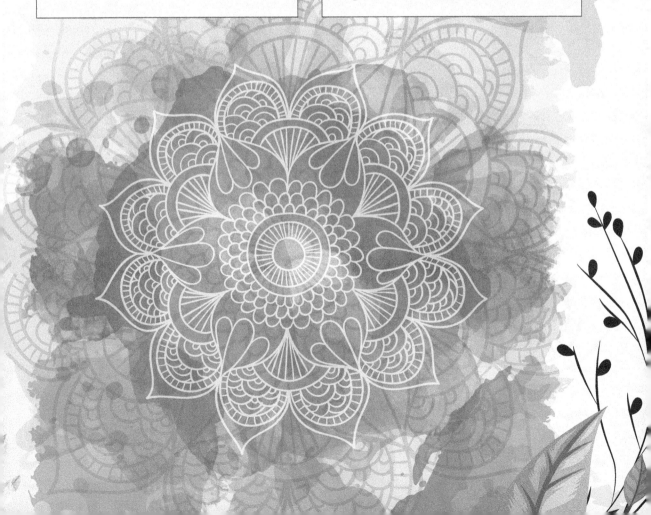

Journal

What I learned about myself this season and how I will bring this wisdom with me.

....

....

....

....

....

....

....

....

....

....

....

....

....

May

TO DO:

-
-
-
-
-
-
-
-
-
-
-
-
-

SUNDAY	MONDAY	TUESDAY
☐	☐	☐
2 Blossom	3	4
9	10	11
16	17	18 Elevate
23	24	25
30	31	☐

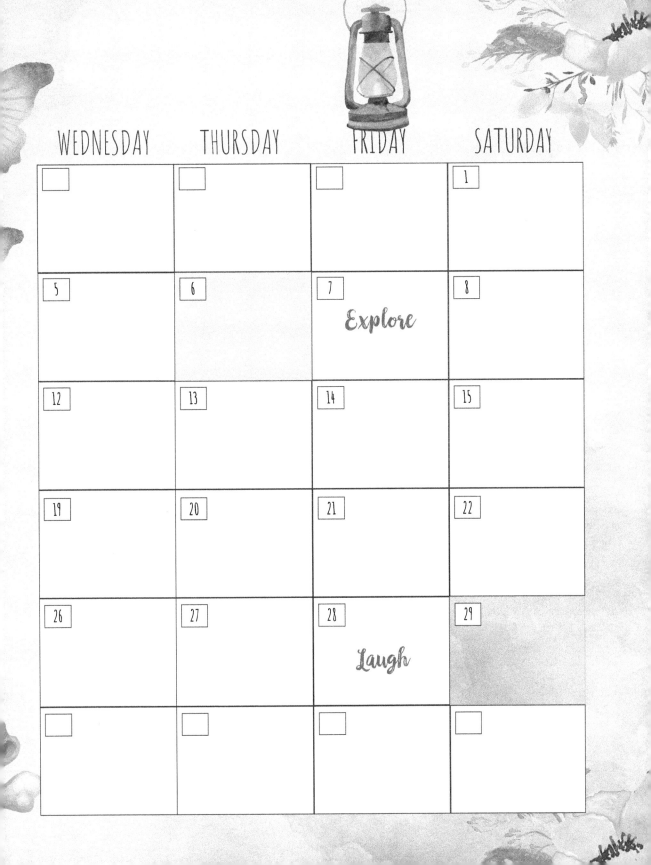

WEDNESDAY	THURSDAY	FRIDAY	SATURDAY
☐	☐	☐	1
5	6	7 *Explore*	8
12	13	14	15
19	20	21	22
26	27	28 *Laugh*	29
☐	☐	☐	☐

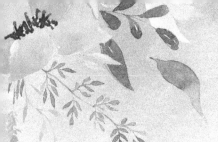

I am loved.

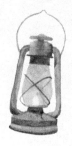

MONDAY	TUESDAY	WEDNESDAY
April 26	April 27	April 28

☐ .... ☐ .... ☐ ....

☐ .... ☐ .... ☐ ....

☐ .... ☐ .... ☐ ....

☐ .... ☐ .... ☐ ....

☐ .... ☐ .... ☐ ....

☐ .... ☐ .... ☐ ....

☐ .... ☐ .... ☐ ....

☐ .... ☐ .... ☐ ....

☐ .... ☐ .... ☐ ....

☐ .... ☐ .... ☐ ....

☐ .... ☐ .... ☐ ....

☐ .... ☐ .... ☐ ....

☐ .... ☐ .... ☐ ....

☐ .... ☐ .... ☐ ....

My movement schedule this week: Monday _____ Tuesday _____
Wednesday _____ Thursday _____ Friday _____
Sat/Sunday _____
The healthy meal I'm most excited about this week is: _____.

THURSDAY

APRIL 29

☐ ....
☐ ....
☐ ....
☐ ....
☐ ....
☐ ....
☐ ....
☐ ....
☐ ....
☐ ....
☐ ....
☐ ....
☐ ....
☐ ....

FRIDAY

APRIL 30

☐ ....
☐ ....
☐ ....
☐ ....
☐ ....
☐ ....
☐ ....
☐ ....
☐ ....
☐ ....
☐ ....
☐ ....
☐ ....
☐ ....

WEEKEND

MAY 1-2

☐ ....
☐ ....
☐ ....
☐ ....
☐ ....
☐ ....
☐ ....
☐ ....
☐ ....
☐ ....
☐ ....
☐ ....
☐ ....
☐ ....

I am hopeful.

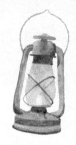

MONDAY	TUESDAY	WEDNESDAY
May 3	May 4	May 5
☐	☐	☐ ....
☐	☐	☐ ....
☐	☐	☐ ....
☐	☐	☐ ....
☐	☐	☐ ....
☐	☐	☐ ....
☐	☐	☐ ....
☐	☐	☐ ....
☐	☐	☐ ....
☐	☐	☐ ....
☐	☐	☐ ....
☐	☐	☐ ....
☐	☐	☐ ....

My movement schedule this week: Monday _____ Tuesday _____

Wednesday _____ Thursday _____ Friday _____

Sat/Sunday _____

The healthy meal I'm most excited about this week is: _____.

THURSDAY
MAY 6

☐ ....
☐ ....
☐ ....
☐ ....
☐ ....
☐ ....
☐ ....
☐ ....
☐ ....
☐ ....
☐ ....
☐ ....
☐ ....
☐ ....

FRIDAY
MAY 7

☐ ....
☐ ....
☐ ....
☐ ....
☐ ....
☐ ....
☐ ....
☐ ....
☐ ....
☐ ....
☐ ....
☐ ....
☐ ....

WEEKEND
MAY 8-9

☐ ....
☐ ....
☐ ....
☐ ....
☐ ....
☐ ....
☐ ....
☐ ....
☐ ....
☐ ....
☐ ....
☐ ....
☐ ....

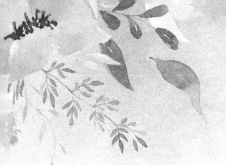

I am kind.

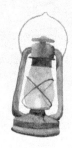

MONDAY	TUESDAY	WEDNESDAY
May 10	May 11	May 12

MONDAY — May 10
- ☐ ....
- ☐ ....
- ☐ ....
- ☐ ....
- ☐ ....
- ☐ ....
- ☐ ....
- ☐ ....
- ☐ ....
- ☐ ....
- ☐ ....
- ☐ ....
- ☐ ....
- ☐ ....

TUESDAY — May 11
- ☐ ....
- ☐ ....
- ☐ ....
- ☐ ....
- ☐ ....
- ☐ ....
- ☐ ....
- ☐ ....
- ☐ ....
- ☐ ....
- ☐ ....
- ☐ ....
- ☐ ....
- ☐ ....

WEDNESDAY — May 12
- ☐ ....
- ☐ ....
- ☐ ....
- ☐ ....
- ☐ ....
- ☐ ....
- ☐ ....
- ☐ ....
- ☐ ....
- ☐ ....
- ☐ ....
- ☐ ....
- ☐ ....
- ☐ ....

My movement schedule this week: Monday _____ Tuesday _____
Wednesday _____ Thursday _____ Friday _____
Sat/Sunday _____
The healthy meal I'm most excited about this week is: _____.

THURSDAY

MAY 13

- ☐ ....
- ☐ ....
- ☐ ....
- ☐ ....
- ☐ ....
- ☐ ....
- ☐ ....
- ☐ ....
- ☐ ....
- ☐ ....
- ☐ ....
- ☐ ....
- ☐ ....
- ☐ ....

FRIDAY

MAY 14

- ☐ ....
- ☐ ....
- ☐ ....
- ☐ ....
- ☐ ....
- ☐ ....
- ☐ ....
- ☐ ....
- ☐ ....
- ☐ ....
- ☐ ....
- ☐ ....
- ☐ ....
- ☐ ....

WEEKEND

MAY 15-16

- ☐ ....
- ☐ ....
- ☐ ....
- ☐ ....
- ☐ ....
- ☐ ....
- ☐ ....
- ☐ ....
- ☐ ....
- ☐ ....
- ☐ ....
- ☐ ....
- ☐ ....
- ☐ ....

I am worthy.

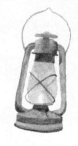

MONDAY	TUESDAY	WEDNESDAY
May 17	May 18	May 19

MONDAY — May 17
- ☐ ....
- ☐ ....
- ☐ ....
- ☐ ....
- ☐ ....
- ☐ ....
- ☐ ....
- ☐ ....
- ☐ ....
- ☐ ....
- ☐ ....
- ☐ ....
- ☐ ....

TUESDAY — May 18
- ☐ ....
- ☐ ....
- ☐ ....
- ☐ ....
- ☐ ....
- ☐ ....
- ☐ ....
- ☐ ....
- ☐ ....
- ☐ ....
- ☐ ....
- ☐ ....
- ☐ ....

WEDNESDAY — May 19
- ☐ ....
- ☐ ....
- ☐ ....
- ☐ ....
- ☐ ....
- ☐ ....
- ☐ ....
- ☐ ....
- ☐ ....
- ☐ ....
- ☐ ....
- ☐ ....
- ☐ ....

My movement schedule this week: Monday _____ Tuesday _____
Wednesday _____ Thursday _____ Friday _____
Sat/Sunday _____
The healthy meal I'm most excited about this week is: _____.

THURSDAY

MAY 20

☐ ....
☐ ....
☐ ....
☐ ....
☐ ....
☐ ....
☐ ....
☐ ....
☐ ....
☐ ....
☐ ....
☐ ....
☐ ....
☐ ....

FRIDAY

MAY 21

☐ ....
☐ ....
☐ ....
☐ ....
☐ ....
☐ ....
☐ ....
☐ ....
☐ ....
☐ ....
☐ ....
☐ ....
☐ ....
☐ ....

WEEKEND

MAY 22-23

☐ ....
☐ ....
☐ ....
☐ ....
☐ ....
☐ ....
☐ ....
☐ ....
☐ ....
☐ ....
☐ ....
☐ ....

I am growing.

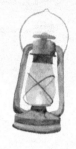

MONDAY	TUESDAY	WEDNESDAY
May 24	May 25	May 26

My movement schedule this week: Monday _____ Tuesday _____
Wednesday _____ Thursday _____ Friday _____
Sat/Sunday _____
The healthy meal I'm most excited about this week is: _____.

THURSDAY

May 27

- ☐ ....
- ☐ ....
- ☐ ....
- ☐ ....
- ☐ ....
- ☐ ....
- ☐ ....
- ☐ ....
- ☐ ....
- ☐ ....
- ☐ ....
- ☐ ....
- ☐ ....
- ☐ ....

FRIDAY

May 28

- ☐ ....
- ☐ ....
- ☐ ....
- ☐ ....
- ☐ ....
- ☐ ....
- ☐ ....
- ☐ ....
- ☐ ....
- ☐ ....
- ☐ ....
- ☐ ....
- ☐ ....
- ☐ ....

WEEKEND

May 29-30

- ☐ ....
- ☐ ....
- ☐ ....
- ☐ ....
- ☐ ....
- ☐ ....
- ☐ ....
- ☐ ....
- ☐ ....
- ☐ ....
- ☐ ....
- ☐ ....
- ☐ ....

I am learning.

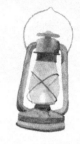

MONDAY	TUESDAY	WEDNESDAY
May 31	June 1	June 2

MONDAY — May 31
- ☐ ....
- ☐ ....
- ☐ ....
- ☐ ....
- ☐ ....
- ☐ ....
- ☐ ....
- ☐ ....
- ☐ ....
- ☐ ....
- ☐ ....
- ☐ ....
- ☐ ....
- ☐ ....

TUESDAY — June 1
- ☐ ....
- ☐ ....
- ☐ ....
- ☐ ....
- ☐ ....
- ☐ ....
- ☐ ....
- ☐ ....
- ☐ ....
- ☐ ....
- ☐ ....
- ☐ ....
- ☐ ....
- ☐ ....

WEDNESDAY — June 2
- ☐ ....
- ☐ ....
- ☐ ....
- ☐ ....
- ☐ ....
- ☐ ....
- ☐ ....
- ☐ ....
- ☐ ....
- ☐ ....
- ☐ ....
- ☐ ....
- ☐ ....
- ☐ ....

Journal

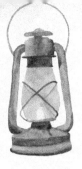

What I learned about myself this season and how
I will bring this wisdom with me.

....

....

....

....

....

....

....

....

....

....

....

....

....

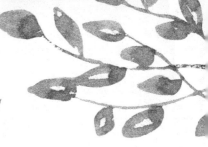

Pitta Season

PITTA/SUMMER *(ruling elements: fire & water) During the summer the atmosphere is hot and moist. People are prone towards heartburn, acid reflux, skin sensitivities, irritability, and impatience.*

THE REMEDY

- [ ] Cool & Refresh
- [ ] Spend time near the water. Swim in the ocean or lakes.
- [ ] Take a vacation.
- [ ] Use lemongrass, sandalwood, or peppermint essential oil.
- [ ] Drink coconut water and aloe vera juice.
- [ ] Avoid spicy & acidic foods.
- [ ] Lay low on hot yoga and competitive sports.
- [ ] Try Yin Yoga to unwind.
- [ ] Make sure to eat so as not to get "hangry".
- [ ] Give yourself a sweet and cooling self-massage with coconut oil and a drop of lavender before showering.

NUTRITION

for Pitta Season

Avoid spicy and acidic foods like tomatoes, garlic, onion, dairy, red meat, vinegar, citrus, excess coffee & excess alcohol. Eat lots of cooling leafy greens, coconuts, watermelon, and sweet vegetables like carrots and sweet potatoes. Be sure to have fats & protein with meals as to avoid hunger pangs. According to Ayurveda, summer is the only time where it's appropriate to eat cold or raw foods. Feel free to add cilantro and mint to your meals to cool off even more.

....

....

....

....

....

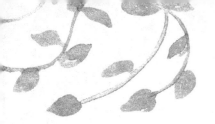

June

TO DO:	SUNDAY	MONDAY	TUESDAY
●	☐	☐	1
●	6	7	8
●			
●	13	14 *Relax*	15
●			
●			
●	20	21	22
●			
●			
●	27 *Self-care*	28	29
●			
●			
●			

WEDNESDAY	THURSDAY	FRIDAY	SATURDAY
2	3	4	5
9	10	11	12 Love
16	17	18	19
23	24 Meditate	25	26
30			

I am chill like a cool breeze.

MONDAY	TUESDAY	WEDNESDAY
May 31	June 1	June 2

MONDAY — May 31
- ☐ ....
- ☐ ....
- ☐ ....
- ☐ ....
- ☐ ....
- ☐ ....
- ☐ ....
- ☐ ....
- ☐ ....
- ☐ ....
- ☐ ....
- ☐ ....
- ☐ ....

TUESDAY — June 1
- ☐ ....
- ☐ ....
- ☐ ....
- ☐ ....
- ☐ ....
- ☐ ....
- ☐ ....
- ☐ ....
- ☐ ....
- ☐ ....
- ☐ ....
- ☐ ....
- ☐ ....

WEDNESDAY — June 2
- ☐ ....
- ☐ ....
- ☐ ....
- ☐ ....
- ☐ ....
- ☐ ....
- ☐ ....
- ☐ ....
- ☐ ....
- ☐ ....
- ☐ ....
- ☐ ....
- ☐ ....

Nutrition: I commit to _____ this week. (example: I commit to brining a balanced lunch to work every day this week.)

Self-Care: I commit to _____ this week. (example: putting lemongrass oil in my diffusor at the office this week).

THURSDAY

June 3

- [ ] ....
- [ ] ....
- [ ] ....
- [ ] ....
- [ ] ....
- [ ] ....
- [ ] ....
- [ ] ....
- [ ] ....
- [ ] ....
- [ ] ....
- [ ] ....
- [ ] ....

FRIDAY

June 4

- [ ] ....
- [ ] ....
- [ ] ....
- [ ] ....
- [ ] ....
- [ ] ....
- [ ] ....
- [ ] ....
- [ ] ....
- [ ] ....
- [ ] ....
- [ ] ....
- [ ] ....

WEEKEND

June 5-6

- [ ] ....
- [ ] ....
- [ ] ....
- [ ] ....
- [ ] ....
- [ ] ....
- [ ] ....
- [ ] ....
- [ ] ....
- [ ] ....
- [ ] ....
- [ ] ....
- [ ] ....

I am blissful.

MONDAY	TUESDAY	WEDNESDAY
June 7	June 8	June 9

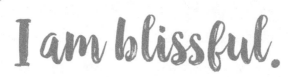

Nutrition: I commit to _____ *this week. (example: I commit to brining a balanced lunch to work every day this week.)*

Self-Care: I commit to _____ *this week. (example: putting lemongrass oil in my diffusor at the office this week).*

THURSDAY
June 10

- [ ] ....
- [ ] ....
- [ ] ....
- [ ] ....
- [ ] ....
- [ ] ....
- [ ] ....
- [ ] ....
- [ ] ....
- [ ] ....
- [ ] ....
- [ ] ....
- [ ] ....
- [ ] ....

FRIDAY
June 11

- [ ] ....
- [ ] ....
- [ ] ....
- [ ] ....
- [ ] ....
- [ ] ....
- [ ] ....
- [ ] ....
- [ ] ....
- [ ] ....
- [ ] ....
- [ ] ....
- [ ] ....
- [ ] ....

WEEKEND
June 12-13

- [ ] ....
- [ ] ....
- [ ] ....
- [ ] ....
- [ ] ....
- [ ] ....
- [ ] ....
- [ ] ....
- [ ] ....
- [ ] ....
- [ ] ....
- [ ] ....
- [ ] ....

I am resilient.

MONDAY	TUESDAY	WEDNESDAY
June 14	June 15	June 16

Nutrition: I commit to _____ *this week. (example: I commit to brining a balanced lunch to work every day this week.)*

Self-Care: I commit to _____ *this week. (example: putting lemongrass oil in my diffusor at the office this week).*

THURSDAY	FRIDAY	WEEKEND
June 17	June 18	June 19-20

THURSDAY — June 17
- ☐ ....
- ☐ ....
- ☐ ....
- ☐ ....
- ☐ ....
- ☐ ....
- ☐ ....
- ☐ ....
- ☐ ....
- ☐ ....
- ☐ ....
- ☐ ....
- ☐ ....
- ☐ ....

FRIDAY — June 18
- ☐ ....
- ☐ ....
- ☐ ....
- ☐ ....
- ☐ ....
- ☐ ....
- ☐ ....
- ☐ ....
- ☐ ....
- ☐ ....
- ☐ ....
- ☐ ....
- ☐ ....
- ☐ ....

WEEKEND — June 19-20
- ☐ ....
- ☐ ....
- ☐ ....
- ☐ ....
- ☐ ....
- ☐ ....
- ☐ ....
- ☐ ....
- ☐ ....
- ☐ ....
- ☐ ....
- ☐ ....

I am patient.

MONDAY	TUESDAY	WEDNESDAY
June 21	June 22	June 23

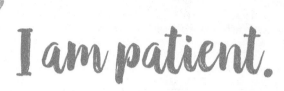

Nutrition: I commit to _____ *this week. (example: I commit to brining a balanced lunch to work every day this week.)*

Self-Care: I commit to _____ *this week. (example: putting lemongrass oil in my diffusor at the office this week).*

THURSDAY	FRIDAY	WEEKEND
June 24	June 25	June 26-27
☐	☐	☐ ....
☐	☐	☐ ....
☐	☐	☐ ....
☐	☐	☐ ....
☐	☐	☐ ....
☐	☐	☐ ....
☐	☐	☐ ....
☐	☐	☐ ....
☐	☐	☐ ....
☐	☐	☐ ....
☐	☐	☐ ....
☐	☐	☐ ....
☐	☐	☐ ....

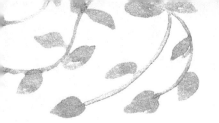
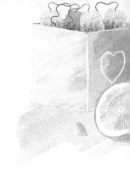

I am whole.

MONDAY

June 28

- [ ] ....
- [ ] ....
- [ ] ....
- [ ] ....
- [ ] ....
- [ ] ....
- [ ] ....
- [ ] ....
- [ ] ....
- [ ] ....
- [ ] ....
- [ ] ....
- [ ] ....
- [ ] ....

TUESDAY

June 29

- [ ] ....
- [ ] ....
- [ ] ....
- [ ] ....
- [ ] ....
- [ ] ....
- [ ] ....
- [ ] ....
- [ ] ....
- [ ] ....
- [ ] ....
- [ ] ....
- [ ] ....
- [ ] ....

WEDNESDAY

June 30

- [ ] ....
- [ ] ....
- [ ] ....
- [ ] ....
- [ ] ....
- [ ] ....
- [ ] ....
- [ ] ....
- [ ] ....
- [ ] ....
- [ ] ....
- [ ] ....
- [ ] ....
- [ ] ....

Journal

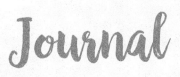

....

....

....

....

....

....

....

....

....

....

....

....

July

TO DO:

- ●
- ●
- ●
- ●
- ●
- ●
- ●
- ●
- ●
- ●
- ●
- ●
- ●

SUNDAY	MONDAY	TUESDAY
☐	☐	☐
4 *Rest*	5	6
11	12	13
18	19	20 *Stretch*
25	26	27

WEDNESDAY	THURSDAY	FRIDAY	SATURDAY
	1 Celebrate (4th)	2	3
7	8	9	10
14	15	16	17
21	22 Chill	23	24
28	29	30	31

I trust the flow of life.

MONDAY	TUESDAY	WEDNESDAY
June 28	June 29	June 30

☐ .... ☐ .... ☐ ....

☐ .... ☐ .... ☐ ....

☐ .... ☐ .... ☐ ....

☐ .... ☐ .... ☐ ....

☐ .... ☐ .... ☐ ....

☐ .... ☐ .... ☐ ....

☐ .... ☐ .... ☐ ....

☐ .... ☐ .... ☐ ....

☐ .... ☐ .... ☐ ....

☐ .... ☐ .... ☐ ....

☐ .... ☐ .... ☐ ....

☐ .... ☐ .... ☐ ....

☐ .... ☐ .... ☐ ....

Nutrition: I commit to _____ *this week. (example: I commit to brining a balanced lunch to work every day this week.)*

Self-Care: I commit to _____ *this week. (example: putting lemongrass oil in my diffusor at the office this week).*

THURSDAY	FRIDAY	WEEKEND
July 1	July 2	July 3-4
☐	☐	☐ ....
☐	☐	☐ ....
☐	☐	☐ ....
☐	☐	☐ ....
☐	☐	☐ ....
☐	☐	☐ ....
☐	☐	☐ ....
☐	☐	☐ ....
☐	☐	☐ ....
☐	☐	☐ ....
☐	☐	☐ ....
☐	☐	☐ ....
☐	☐	☐ ....
☐	☐	☐ ....

I am kind.

MONDAY	TUESDAY	WEDNESDAY
July 5	July 6	July 7

MONDAY — July 5

- ☐ ....
- ☐ ....
- ☐ ....
- ☐ ....
- ☐ ....
- ☐ ....
- ☐ ....
- ☐ ....
- ☐ ....
- ☐ ....
- ☐ ....
- ☐ ....
- ☐ ....

TUESDAY — July 6

- ☐ ....
- ☐ ....
- ☐ ....
- ☐ ....
- ☐ ....
- ☐ ....
- ☐ ....
- ☐ ....
- ☐ ....
- ☐ ....
- ☐ ....
- ☐ ....
- ☐ ....

WEDNESDAY — July 7

- ☐ ....
- ☐ ....
- ☐ ....
- ☐ ....
- ☐ ....
- ☐ ....
- ☐ ....
- ☐ ....
- ☐ ....
- ☐ ....
- ☐ ....
- ☐ ....
- ☐ ....

Nutrition: I commit to _____ this week. (example: I commit to brining a balanced lunch to work every day this week.)

Self-Care: I commit to _____ this week. (example: putting lemongrass oil in my diffusor at the office this week).

THURSDAY	FRIDAY	WEEKEND
July 8	July 9	July 10-11

THURSDAY — July 8
- ☐ ....
- ☐ ....
- ☐ ....
- ☐ ....
- ☐ ....
- ☐ ....
- ☐ ....
- ☐ ....
- ☐ ....
- ☐ ....
- ☐ ....
- ☐ ....
- ☐ ....
- ☐ ....

FRIDAY — July 9
- ☐ ....
- ☐ ....
- ☐ ....
- ☐ ....
- ☐ ....
- ☐ ....
- ☐ ....
- ☐ ....
- ☐ ....
- ☐ ....
- ☐ ....
- ☐ ....
- ☐ ....

WEEKEND — July 10-11
- ☐ ....
- ☐ ....
- ☐ ....
- ☐ ....
- ☐ ....
- ☐ ....
- ☐ ....
- ☐ ....
- ☐ ....
- ☐ ....
- ☐ ....
- ☐ ....
- ☐ ....

I am satisfied.

MONDAY	TUESDAY	WEDNESDAY
July 12	July 13	July 14

MONDAY — July 12
- ☐ ....
- ☐ ....
- ☐ ....
- ☐ ....
- ☐ ....
- ☐ ....
- ☐ ....
- ☐ ....
- ☐ ....
- ☐ ....
- ☐ ....
- ☐ ....
- ☐ ....
- ☐ ....

TUESDAY — July 13
- ☐ ....
- ☐ ....
- ☐ ....
- ☐ ....
- ☐ ....
- ☐ ....
- ☐ ....
- ☐ ....
- ☐ ....
- ☐ ....
- ☐ ....
- ☐ ....
- ☐ ....
- ☐ ....

WEDNESDAY — July 14
- ☐ ....
- ☐ ....
- ☐ ....
- ☐ ....
- ☐ ....
- ☐ ....
- ☐ ....
- ☐ ....
- ☐ ....
- ☐ ....
- ☐ ....
- ☐ ....
- ☐ ....
- ☐ ....

Nutrition: I commit to _____ *this week. (example: I commit to brining a balanced lunch to work every day this week.)*

Self-Care: I commit to _____ *this week. (example: putting lemongrass oil in my diffusor at the office this week).*

THURSDAY	FRIDAY	WEEKEND
July 15	July 16	July 17-18
☐	☐	☐ ....
☐	☐	☐ ....
☐	☐	☐ ....
☐	☐	☐ ....
☐	☐	☐ ....
☐	☐	☐ ....
☐	☐	☐ ....
☐	☐	☐ ....
☐	☐	☐ ....
☐	☐	☐ ....
☐	☐	☐ ....
☐	☐	☐ ....
☐	☐	☐ ....

I am giving myself permission to relax.

MONDAY	TUESDAY	WEDNESDAY
July 19	July 20	July 21

MONDAY — July 19

- ☐ ....
- ☐ ....
- ☐ ....
- ☐ ....
- ☐ ....
- ☐ ....
- ☐ ....
- ☐ ....
- ☐ ....
- ☐ ....
- ☐ ....
- ☐ ....
- ☐ ....

TUESDAY — July 20

- ☐ ....
- ☐ ....
- ☐ ....
- ☐ ....
- ☐ ....
- ☐ ....
- ☐ ....
- ☐ ....
- ☐ ....
- ☐ ....
- ☐ ....
- ☐ ....
- ☐ ....

WEDNESDAY — July 21

- ☐ ....
- ☐ ....
- ☐ ....
- ☐ ....
- ☐ ....
- ☐ ....
- ☐ ....
- ☐ ....
- ☐ ....
- ☐ ....
- ☐ ....
- ☐ ....

Nutrition: I commit to _____ *this week. (example: I commit to brining a balanced lunch to work every day this week.)*

Self-Care: I commit to _____ *this week. (example: putting lemongrass oil in my diffusor at the office this week).*

THURSDAY	FRIDAY	WEEKEND
July 22	July 23	July 24-25
☐	☐	☐ ....
☐	☐	☐ ....
☐	☐	☐ ....
☐	☐	☐ ....
☐	☐	☐ ....
☐	☐	☐ ....
☐	☐	☐ ....
☐	☐	☐ ....
☐	☐	☐ ....
☐	☐	☐ ....
☐	☐	☐ ....
☐	☐	☐ ....
☐	☐	☐ ....

I am enough.

MONDAY	TUESDAY	WEDNESDAY
July 26	July 27	July 28

MONDAY — July 26

- ☐ ....
- ☐ ....
- ☐ ....
- ☐ ....
- ☐ ....
- ☐ ....
- ☐ ....
- ☐ ....
- ☐ ....
- ☐ ....
- ☐ ....
- ☐ ....
- ☐ ....

TUESDAY — July 27

- ☐ ....
- ☐ ....
- ☐ ....
- ☐ ....
- ☐ ....
- ☐ ....
- ☐ ....
- ☐ ....
- ☐ ....
- ☐ ....
- ☐ ....
- ☐ ....
- ☐ ....

WEDNESDAY — July 28

- ☐ ....
- ☐ ....
- ☐ ....
- ☐ ....
- ☐ ....
- ☐ ....
- ☐ ....
- ☐ ....
- ☐ ....
- ☐ ....
- ☐ ....
- ☐ ....
- ☐ ....

Nutrition: I commit to _____ *this week. (example: I commit to brining a balanced lunch to work every day this week.)*

Self-Care: I commit to _____ *this week. (example: putting lemongrass oil in my diffusor at the office this week).*

THURSDAY	FRIDAY	WEEKEND
July 29	July 30	July 31-August 1
☐	☐	☐ ....
☐	☐	☐ ....
☐	☐	☐ ....
☐	☐	☐ ....
☐	☐	☐ ....
☐	☐	☐ ....
☐	☐	☐ ....
☐	☐	☐ ....
☐	☐	☐ ....
☐	☐	☐ ....
☐	☐	☐ ....
☐	☐	☐ ....
☐	☐	☐ ....

SUMMER SALAD

INGREDIENTS

- 1 cup kale
- 1/4 cup dried cranberries
- 1/4 cup pine seeds
- 1/4 cups slices kalamate olives
- salt and pepper to taste
- 1 tablespoon of grape seed oil

DIRECTIONS

Place in ingredients in ziplock bag. Massage the oils into the kale, and shake the ingredients in the bag. Serve on a plat with a few slices of fresh avocado.

COCONUT QUINOA RICE
and Vegetables

INGREDIENTS

- 5 cups mixed vegetables chopped: carrots and broccoli (use any summer vegetable of your choosing)
- 1/2 tablespoon ginger chopped
- 1/2 cup white basmati rice
- 1/2 cup quinoa
- 1 cup coconut milk
- 1 1/2 cups water
- 1/4 cup shredded unsweetened coconut
- Salt to taste

DIRECTIONS

Cook the rice, quinoa, ginger, and vegetables in the coconut milk/water mixture (stovetop or rice cooker) until cooked. In a skillet, dry roast the shredded coconut over low heat until golden brown and fragrant. Add the coconut and salt and gently stir into the coco-nut/rice/quinoa mixture.

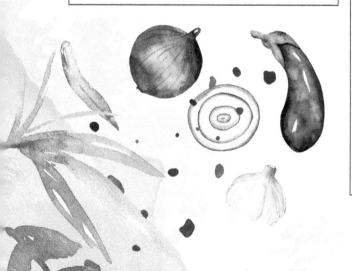

MEAL PREP:

- DANDELION GREENS
- KALE
- COCONUT
- MANGOES
- TOFU
- BASMATI RICE
- AVOCADO
- CUCUMBERS
- SWEET POTATOES
- MINT
- CILANTRO

I'M MAKING:

- COCONUT BASMATI RICE
- SUMMER KALE SALAD
- MANGO SALSA
- SWEET POTATOES WITH PAN- SEARED TOFU
- ☐ ....
- ☐ ....
- ☐ ....
- ☐ ....
- ☐ ....

PITTA STRENGHTS

Ambitious

Charismatic

Organized

Goal Oriented

Leadership

MY STRENGTHS RIGHT NOW:

August

TO DO:

-
-
-
-
-
-
-
-
-
-
-
-
-

SUNDAY	MONDAY	TUESDAY
1	2	3 Breathe
8	9	10
15	16	17
22	23	24
29	30 Kindness	31

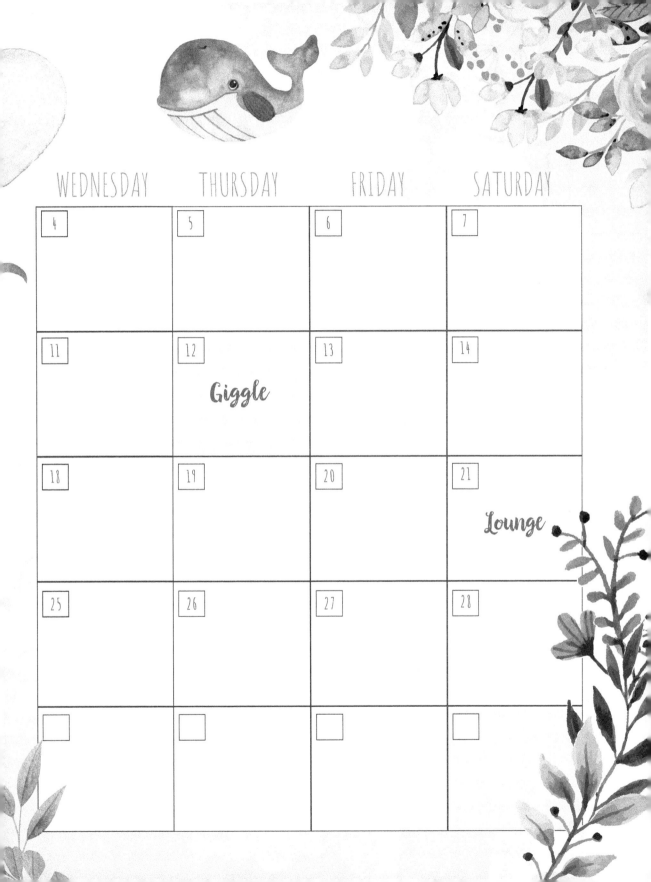

WEDNESDAY	THURSDAY	FRIDAY	SATURDAY
4	5	6	7
11	12 *Giggle*	13	14
18	19	20	21 *Lounge*
25	26	27	28

I am playful.

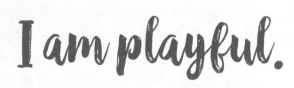

MONDAY	TUESDAY	WEDNESDAY
August 2	August 3	August 4

MONDAY — August 2
- ☐ ....
- ☐ ....
- ☐ ....
- ☐ ....
- ☐ ....
- ☐ ....
- ☐ ....
- ☐ ....
- ☐ ....
- ☐ ....
- ☐ ....
- ☐ ....
- ☐ ....

TUESDAY — August 3
- ☐ ....
- ☐ ....
- ☐ ....
- ☐ ....
- ☐ ....
- ☐ ....
- ☐ ....
- ☐ ....
- ☐ ....
- ☐ ....
- ☐ ....
- ☐ ....
- ☐ ....

WEDNESDAY — August 4
- ☐ ....
- ☐ ....
- ☐ ....
- ☐ ....
- ☐ ....
- ☐ ....
- ☐ ....
- ☐ ....
- ☐ ....
- ☐ ....
- ☐ ....
- ☐ ....
- ☐ ....

THURSDAY

AUGUST 5

☐ ....
☐ ....
☐ ....
☐ ....
☐ ....
☐ ....
☐ ....
☐ ....
☐ ....
☐ ....
☐ ....
☐ ....
☐ ....

FRIDAY

AUGUST 6

☐ ....
☐ ....
☐ ....
☐ ....
☐ ....
☐ ....
☐ ....
☐ ....
☐ ....
☐ ....
☐ ....
☐ ....
☐ ....

WEEKEND

AUGUST 7-8

☐ ....
☐ ....
☐ ....
☐ ....
☐ ....
☐ ....
☐ ....
☐ ....
☐ ....
☐ ....
☐ ....
☐ ....

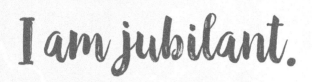

I am jubilant.

MONDAY

August 9

- ☐ ....
- ☐ ....
- ☐ ....
- ☐ ....
- ☐ ....
- ☐ ....
- ☐ ....
- ☐ ....
- ☐ ....
- ☐ ....
- ☐ ....
- ☐ ....
- ☐ ....

TUESDAY

August 10

- ☐ ....
- ☐ ....
- ☐ ....
- ☐ ....
- ☐ ....
- ☐ ....
- ☐ ....
- ☐ ....
- ☐ ....
- ☐ ....
- ☐ ....
- ☐ ....
- ☐ ....

WEDNESDAY

August 11

- ☐ ....
- ☐ ....
- ☐ ....
- ☐ ....
- ☐ ....
- ☐ ....
- ☐ ....
- ☐ ....
- ☐ ....
- ☐ ....
- ☐ ....
- ☐ ....
- ☐ ....

Nutrition: I commit to _____ this week. (example: I commit to brining a balanced lunch to work every day this week.)

Self-Care: I commit to _____ this week. (example: putting lemongrass oil in my diffusor at the office this week).

THURSDAY	FRIDAY	WEEKEND
AUGUST 12	AUGUST 13	AUGUST 14-15

THURSDAY — August 12

- [ ] ....
- [ ] ....
- [ ] ....
- [ ] ....
- [ ] ....
- [ ] ....
- [ ] ....
- [ ] ....
- [ ] ....
- [ ] ....
- [ ] ....
- [ ] ....
- [ ] ....
- [ ] ....

FRIDAY — August 13

- [ ] ....
- [ ] ....
- [ ] ....
- [ ] ....
- [ ] ....
- [ ] ....
- [ ] ....
- [ ] ....
- [ ] ....
- [ ] ....
- [ ] ....
- [ ] ....
- [ ] ....
- [ ] ....

WEEKEND — August 14-15

- [ ] ....
- [ ] ....
- [ ] ....
- [ ] ....
- [ ] ....
- [ ] ....
- [ ] ....
- [ ] ....
- [ ] ....
- [ ] ....
- [ ] ....
- [ ] ....
- [ ] ....

I am unwinding.

MONDAY	TUESDAY	WEDNESDAY
August 16	August 17	August 18

MONDAY — August 16

- ☐ ....
- ☐ ....
- ☐ ....
- ☐ ....
- ☐ ....
- ☐ ....
- ☐ ....
- ☐ ....
- ☐ ....
- ☐ ....
- ☐ ....
- ☐ ....
- ☐ ....

TUESDAY — August 17

- ☐ ....
- ☐ ....
- ☐ ....
- ☐ ....
- ☐ ....
- ☐ ....
- ☐ ....
- ☐ ....
- ☐ ....
- ☐ ....
- ☐ ....
- ☐ ....
- ☐ ....

WEDNESDAY — August 18

- ☐ ....
- ☐ ....
- ☐ ....
- ☐ ....
- ☐ ....
- ☐ ....
- ☐ ....
- ☐ ....
- ☐ ....
- ☐ ....
- ☐ ....
- ☐ ....
- ☐ ....

Nutrition: I commit to _____ *this week. (example: I commit to brining a balanced lunch to work every day this week.)*

Self-Care: I commit to _____ *this week. (example: putting lemongrass oil in my diffusor at the office this week).*

THURSDAY	FRIDAY	WEEKEND
August 19	August 20	August 21-22

THURSDAY — August 19

- ☐ ....
- ☐ ....
- ☐ ....
- ☐ ....
- ☐ ....
- ☐ ....
- ☐ ....
- ☐ ....
- ☐ ....
- ☐ ....
- ☐ ....
- ☐ ....
- ☐ ....

FRIDAY — August 20

- ☐ ....
- ☐ ....
- ☐ ....
- ☐ ....
- ☐ ....
- ☐ ....
- ☐ ....
- ☐ ....
- ☐ ....
- ☐ ....
- ☐ ....
- ☐ ....
- ☐ ....

WEEKEND — August 21-22

- ☐ ....
- ☐ ....
- ☐ ....
- ☐ ....
- ☐ ....
- ☐ ....
- ☐ ....
- ☐ ....
- ☐ ....
- ☐ ....
- ☐ ....
- ☐ ....

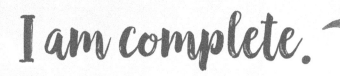

I am complete.

MONDAY	TUESDAY	WEDNESDAY
AUGUST 23	AUGUST 24	AUGUST 25
☐	☐	☐ ....
☐	☐	☐ ....
☐	☐	☐ ....
☐	☐	☐ ....
☐	☐	☐ ....
☐	☐	☐ ....
☐	☐	☐ ....
☐	☐	☐ ....
☐	☐	☐ ....
☐	☐	☐ ....
☐	☐	☐ ....
☐	☐	☐ ....
☐	☐	☐ ....
☐	☐	☐ ....

Nutrition: I commit to _____ *this week. (example: I commit to brining a balanced lunch to work every day this week.)*

Self-Care: I commit to _____ *this week. (example: putting lemongrass oil in my diffusor at the office this week).*

THURSDAY	FRIDAY	WEEKEND
AUGUST 26	AUGUST 27	AUGUST 28-29

THURSDAY

AUGUST 26

- ☐ ....
- ☐ ....
- ☐ ....
- ☐ ....
- ☐ ....
- ☐ ....
- ☐ ....
- ☐ ....
- ☐ ....
- ☐ ....
- ☐ ....
- ☐ ....
- ☐ ....

FRIDAY

AUGUST 27

- ☐ ....
- ☐ ....
- ☐ ....
- ☐ ....
- ☐ ....
- ☐ ....
- ☐ ....
- ☐ ....
- ☐ ....
- ☐ ....
- ☐ ....
- ☐ ....
- ☐ ....

WEEKEND

AUGUST 28-29

- ☐ ....
- ☐ ....
- ☐ ....
- ☐ ....
- ☐ ....
- ☐ ....
- ☐ ....
- ☐ ....
- ☐ ....
- ☐ ....
- ☐ ....
- ☐ ....
- ☐ ....

I am delighted.

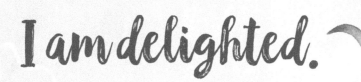

MONDAY	TUESDAY	WEDNESDAY
August 30	August 31	September 1

MONDAY — August 30

- ☐ ....
- ☐ ....
- ☐ ....
- ☐ ....
- ☐ ....
- ☐ ....
- ☐ ....
- ☐ ....
- ☐ ....
- ☐ ....
- ☐ ....
- ☐ ....
- ☐ ....

TUESDAY — August 31

- ☐ ....
- ☐ ....
- ☐ ....
- ☐ ....
- ☐ ....
- ☐ ....
- ☐ ....
- ☐ ....
- ☐ ....
- ☐ ....
- ☐ ....
- ☐ ....
- ☐ ....

WEDNESDAY — September 1

- ☐ ....
- ☐ ....
- ☐ ....
- ☐ ....
- ☐ ....
- ☐ ....
- ☐ ....
- ☐ ....
- ☐ ....
- ☐ ....
- ☐ ....
- ☐ ....
- ☐ ....

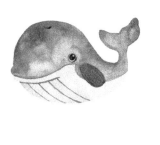

Journal

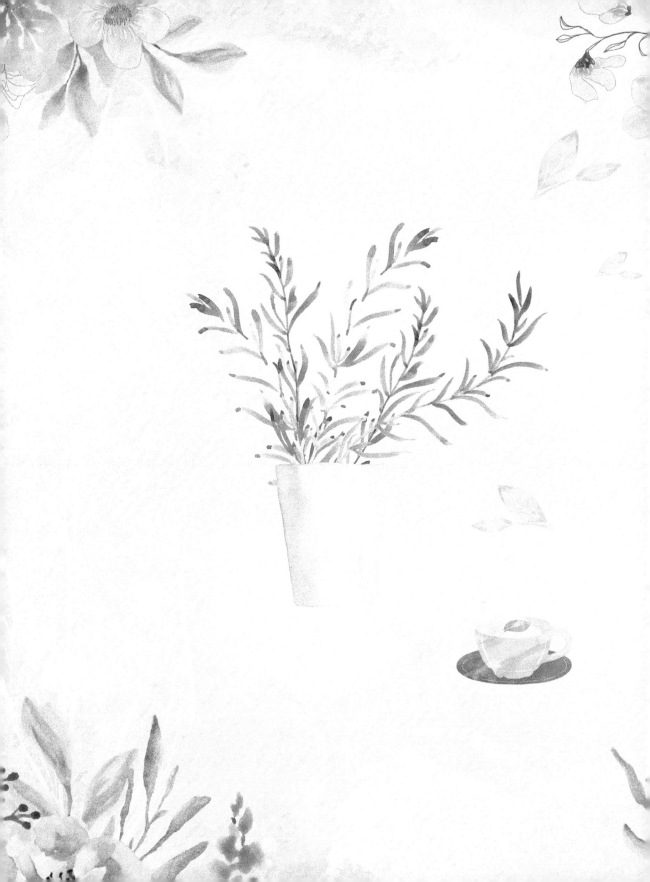

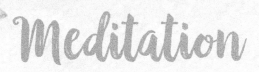

Meditation

THE GLAD MEDITATION

Today I am Grateful for

....

Today I Learned

....

Today I Accomplished

....

Today I was Delighted by

....

GUIDED MEDITATION

Metta, Loving-Kindness Meditations on Insight Timer

September

TO DO:

- ○
- ○
- ○
- ○
- ○
- ○
- ○
- ○
- ○
- ○
- ○
- ○
- ○

SUNDAY	MONDAY	TUESDAY
☐	☐	☐
5	6 *Transitioning*	7
12	13	14
19	20	21 *Slowing Down*
26	27	28

WEDNESDAY	THURSDAY	FRIDAY	SATURDAY
1	2 *Cooling Down*	3	4
8	9	10	11
15	16	17	18
22	23 *Believe*	24	25
29	30		

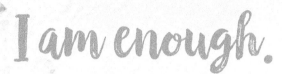

I am enough.

MONDAY	TUESDAY	WEDNESDAY
AUGUST 30	AUGUST 31	SEPTEMBER 1

MONDAY — AUGUST 30

- ☐ ....
- ☐ ....
- ☐ ....
- ☐ ....
- ☐ ....
- ☐ ....
- ☐ ....
- ☐ ....
- ☐ ....
- ☐ ....
- ☐ ....
- ☐ ....
- ☐ ....
- ☐ ....

TUESDAY — AUGUST 31

- ☐ ....
- ☐ ....
- ☐ ....
- ☐ ....
- ☐ ....
- ☐ ....
- ☐ ....
- ☐ ....
- ☐ ....
- ☐ ....
- ☐ ....
- ☐ ....
- ☐ ....
- ☐ ....

WEDNESDAY — SEPTEMBER 1

- ☐ ....
- ☐ ....
- ☐ ....
- ☐ ....
- ☐ ....
- ☐ ....
- ☐ ....
- ☐ ....
- ☐ ....
- ☐ ....
- ☐ ....
- ☐ ....
- ☐ ....
- ☐ ....

Nutrition: I commit to _____ *this week. (example: I commit to brining a balanced lunch to work every day this week.)*

Self-Care: I commit to _____ *this week. (example: putting lemongrass oil in my diffusor at the office this week).*

THURSDAY

September 2

- ☐ ....
- ☐ ....
- ☐ ....
- ☐ ....
- ☐ ....
- ☐ ....
- ☐ ....
- ☐ ....
- ☐ ....
- ☐ ....
- ☐ ....
- ☐ ....
- ☐ ....
- ☐ ....

FRIDAY

September 3

- ☐ ....
- ☐ ....
- ☐ ....
- ☐ ....
- ☐ ....
- ☐ ....
- ☐ ....
- ☐ ....
- ☐ ....
- ☐ ....
- ☐ ....
- ☐ ....
- ☐ ....
- ☐ ....

WEEKEND

September 4-5

- ☐ ....
- ☐ ....
- ☐ ....
- ☐ ....
- ☐ ....
- ☐ ....
- ☐ ....
- ☐ ....
- ☐ ....
- ☐ ....
- ☐ ....
- ☐ ....
- ☐ ....
- ☐ ....

I am honest.

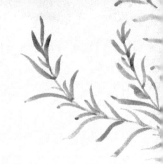

MONDAY	TUESDAY	WEDNESDAY
September 6	September 7	September 8

MONDAY — September 6
- ☐ ....
- ☐ ....
- ☐ ....
- ☐ ....
- ☐ ....
- ☐ ....
- ☐ ....
- ☐ ....
- ☐ ....
- ☐ ....
- ☐ ....
- ☐ ....
- ☐ ....
- ☐ ....

TUESDAY — September 7
- ☐ ....
- ☐ ....
- ☐ ....
- ☐ ....
- ☐ ....
- ☐ ....
- ☐ ....
- ☐ ....
- ☐ ....
- ☐ ....
- ☐ ....
- ☐ ....
- ☐ ....
- ☐ ....

WEDNESDAY — September 8
- ☐ ....
- ☐ ....
- ☐ ....
- ☐ ....
- ☐ ....
- ☐ ....
- ☐ ....
- ☐ ....
- ☐ ....
- ☐ ....
- ☐ ....
- ☐ ....
- ☐ ....
- ☐ ....

Nutrition: I commit to _____ *this week. (example: I commit to brining a balanced lunch to work every day this week.)*

Self-Care: I commit to _____ *this week. (example: putting lemongrass oil in my diffusor at the office this week).*

THURSDAY	FRIDAY	WEEKEND
September 9	September 10	September 11-12

☐ ....
☐ ....
☐ ....
☐ ....
☐ ....
☐ ....
☐ ....
☐ ....
☐ ....
☐ ....
☐ ....
☐ ....
☐ ....

I am capable.

MONDAY	TUESDAY	WEDNESDAY
September 13	September 14	September 15

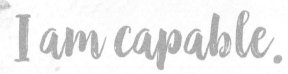

MONDAY

September 13

☐ ....
☐ ....
☐ ....
☐ ....
☐ ....
☐ ....
☐ ....
☐ ....
☐ ....
☐ ....
☐ ....
☐ ....
☐ ....
☐ ....

TUESDAY

September 14

☐ ....
☐ ....
☐ ....
☐ ....
☐ ....
☐ ....
☐ ....
☐ ....
☐ ....
☐ ....
☐ ....
☐ ....
☐ ....
☐ ....

WEDNESDAY

September 15

☐ ....
☐ ....
☐ ....
☐ ....
☐ ....
☐ ....
☐ ....
☐ ....
☐ ....
☐ ....
☐ ....
☐ ....
☐ ....
☐ ....

Nutrition: I commit to _____ this week. (example: I commit to brining a balanced lunch to work every day this week.)

Self-Care: I commit to _____ this week. (example: putting lemongrass oil in my diffusor at the office this week).

THURSDAY

September 16

- [ ] ....
- [ ] ....
- [ ] ....
- [ ] ....
- [ ] ....
- [ ] ....
- [ ] ....
- [ ] ....
- [ ] ....
- [ ] ....
- [ ] ....
- [ ] ....
- [ ] ....
- [ ] ....

FRIDAY

September 17

- [ ] ....
- [ ] ....
- [ ] ....
- [ ] ....
- [ ] ....
- [ ] ....
- [ ] ....
- [ ] ....
- [ ] ....
- [ ] ....
- [ ] ....
- [ ] ....
- [ ] ....

WEEKEND

September 18-19

- [ ] ....
- [ ] ....
- [ ] ....
- [ ] ....
- [ ] ....
- [ ] ....
- [ ] ....
- [ ] ....
- [ ] ....
- [ ] ....
- [ ] ....
- [ ] ....

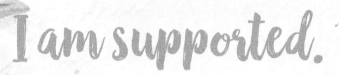

I am supported.

MONDAY	TUESDAY	WEDNESDAY
September 20	September 21	September 22

MONDAY — September 20
- ☐ ....
- ☐ ....
- ☐ ....
- ☐ ....
- ☐ ....
- ☐ ....
- ☐ ....
- ☐ ....
- ☐ ....
- ☐ ....
- ☐ ....
- ☐ ....
- ☐ ....

TUESDAY — September 21
- ☐ ....
- ☐ ....
- ☐ ....
- ☐ ....
- ☐ ....
- ☐ ....
- ☐ ....
- ☐ ....
- ☐ ....
- ☐ ....
- ☐ ....
- ☐ ....
- ☐ ....

WEDNESDAY — September 22
- ☐ ....
- ☐ ....
- ☐ ....
- ☐ ....
- ☐ ....
- ☐ ....
- ☐ ....
- ☐ ....
- ☐ ....
- ☐ ....
- ☐ ....
- ☐ ....
- ☐ ....

Nutrition: I commit to _____ *this week. (example: I commit to brining a balanced lunch to work every day this week.)*

Self-Care: I commit to _____ *this week. (example: putting lemongrass oil in my diffusor at the office this week).*

THURSDAY	**FRIDAY**	**WEEKEND**
September 23	September 24	September 25-26

Thursday — September 23

☐ ....
☐ ....
☐ ....
☐ ....
☐ ....
☐ ....
☐ ....
☐ ....
☐ ....
☐ ....
☐ ....
☐ ....
☐ ....

Friday — September 24

☐ ....
☐ ....
☐ ....
☐ ....
☐ ....
☐ ....
☐ ....
☐ ....
☐ ....
☐ ....
☐ ....
☐ ....
☐ ....

Weekend — September 25-26

☐ ....
☐ ....
☐ ....
☐ ....
☐ ....
☐ ....
☐ ....
☐ ....
☐ ....
☐ ....
☐ ....
☐ ....
☐ ....

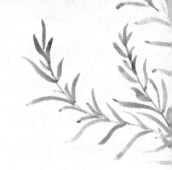

I am strong.

MONDAY

September 27

- ☐ ....
- ☐ ....
- ☐ ....
- ☐ ....
- ☐ ....
- ☐ ....
- ☐ ....
- ☐ ....
- ☐ ....
- ☐ ....
- ☐ ....
- ☐ ....
- ☐ ....

TUESDAY

September 28

- ☐ ....
- ☐ ....
- ☐ ....
- ☐ ....
- ☐ ....
- ☐ ....
- ☐ ....
- ☐ ....
- ☐ ....
- ☐ ....
- ☐ ....
- ☐ ....
- ☐ ....

WEDNESDAY

September 29

- ☐ ....
- ☐ ....
- ☐ ....
- ☐ ....
- ☐ ....
- ☐ ....
- ☐ ....
- ☐ ....
- ☐ ....
- ☐ ....
- ☐ ....
- ☐ ....
- ☐ ....

Nutrition: I commit to _____ *this week. (example: I commit to brining a balanced lunch to work every day this week.)*

Self-Care: I commit to _____ *this week. (example: putting lemongrass oil in my diffusor at the office this week).*

THURSDAY	FRIDAY	WEEKEND
September 30	October 1	October 2-3

THURSDAY — September 30

- ☐ ....
- ☐ ....
- ☐ ....
- ☐ ....
- ☐ ....
- ☐ ....
- ☐ ....
- ☐ ....
- ☐ ....
- ☐ ....
- ☐ ....
- ☐ ....
- ☐ ....
- ☐ ....

FRIDAY — October 1

- ☐ ....
- ☐ ....
- ☐ ....
- ☐ ....
- ☐ ....
- ☐ ....
- ☐ ....
- ☐ ....
- ☐ ....
- ☐ ....
- ☐ ....
- ☐ ....
- ☐ ....
- ☐ ....

WEEKEND — October 2-3

- ☐ ....
- ☐ ....
- ☐ ....
- ☐ ....
- ☐ ....
- ☐ ....
- ☐ ....
- ☐ ....
- ☐ ....
- ☐ ....
- ☐ ....
- ☐ ....
- ☐ ....
- ☐ ....

Journal

Write a supportive letter to yourself. As though you were writing to someone you love most in the world; acknowledge your strengths and positive qualities, offer support, and guidance, and above all, tell yourself how loved you are.

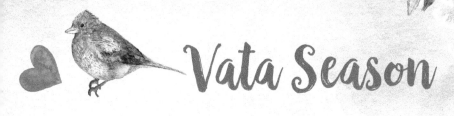

Vata Season

OCTOBER: *The beginning of Vata Season. Remember to slow down. Ground. Take time for Self-Care. Return to warm, moist, and spiced foods such as sweet potato chili, pumpkin spiced oatmeal, and dates sprinkled with cardamom.*

MEDITATION

> *Breathing through the nose— Inhale for 4-3-2-1. Hold the breath. Exhale 4-3-2-1. Repeat this 3x morning and night.*

GUIDED MEDITATION

> *Yoga Nidra on Insight Timer. This short guided, progressive relaxation will help calm your nervous system and help you feel more settled and rested.*

BEST TYPES OF MOVEMENT FOR VATA SEASON: *Light weight lifting/strength building, Hatha or Yin Yoga, hiking, and pilates. Nothing too fast or jarring on the joints.*

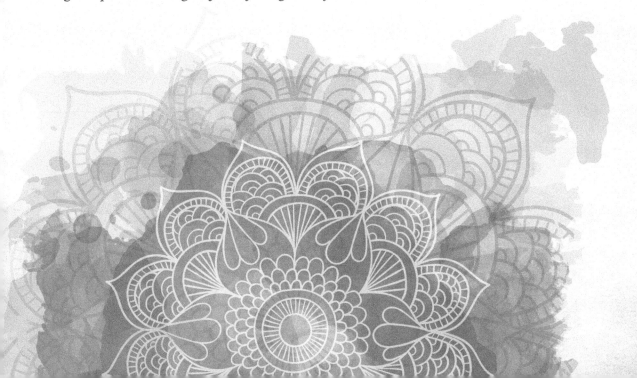

October

TO DO:

- ●
- ●
- ●
- ●
- ●
- ●
- ●
- ●
- ●
- ●
- ●
- ●
- ●

SUNDAY	MONDAY	TUESDAY
☐	☐	☐
3	4	5
10	11	12 Ground
17	18	19
24	25 Nature	26
31	☐	☐

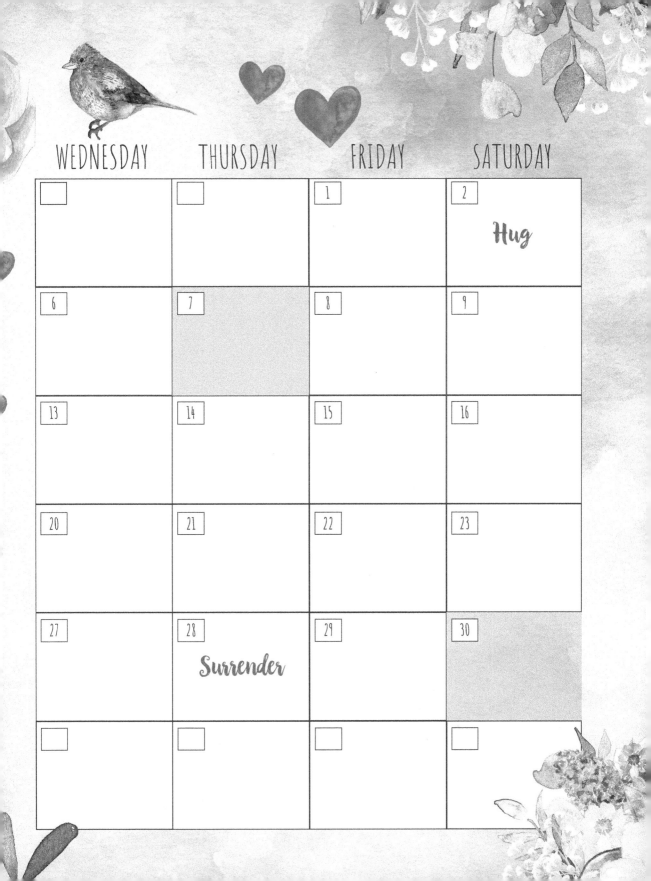

WEDNESDAY	THURSDAY	FRIDAY	SATURDAY
		1	2 *Hug*
6	7	8	9
13	14	15	16
20	21	22	23
27	28 *Surrender*	29	30

I am connected to mother nature.

MONDAY	TUESDAY	WEDNESDAY
September 27	August 28	September 29

MONDAY — September 27

- ☐ ....
- ☐ ....
- ☐ ....
- ☐ ....
- ☐ ....
- ☐ ....
- ☐ ....
- ☐ ....
- ☐ ....
- ☐ ....
- ☐ ....
- ☐ ....
- ☐ ....
- ☐ ....

TUESDAY — August 28

- ☐ ....
- ☐ ....
- ☐ ....
- ☐ ....
- ☐ ....
- ☐ ....
- ☐ ....
- ☐ ....
- ☐ ....
- ☐ ....
- ☐ ....
- ☐ ....
- ☐ ....
- ☐ ....

WEDNESDAY — September 29

- ☐ ....
- ☐ ....
- ☐ ....
- ☐ ....
- ☐ ....
- ☐ ....
- ☐ ....
- ☐ ....
- ☐ ....
- ☐ ....
- ☐ ....
- ☐ ....
- ☐ ....
- ☐ ....

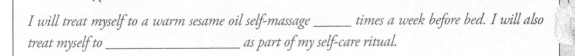

I will treat myself to a warm sesame oil self-massage _____ times a week before bed. I will also treat myself to _____ as part of my self-care ritual.

THURSDAY

September 30

- ☐ ....
- ☐ ....
- ☐ ....
- ☐ ....
- ☐ ....
- ☐ ....
- ☐ ....
- ☐ ....
- ☐ ....
- ☐ ....
- ☐ ....
- ☐ ....
- ☐ ....

FRIDAY

October 1

- ☐ ....
- ☐ ....
- ☐ ....
- ☐ ....
- ☐ ....
- ☐ ....
- ☐ ....
- ☐ ....
- ☐ ....
- ☐ ....
- ☐ ....
- ☐ ....
- ☐ ....

WEEKEND

October 2-3

- ☐ ....
- ☐ ....
- ☐ ....
- ☐ ....
- ☐ ....
- ☐ ....
- ☐ ....
- ☐ ....
- ☐ ....
- ☐ ....
- ☐ ....
- ☐ ....
- ☐ ....

I plant my feet in the earth.

MONDAY	TUESDAY	WEDNESDAY
October 4	October 5	October 6

MONDAY — October 4

- ☐ ....
- ☐ ....
- ☐ ....
- ☐ ....
- ☐ ....
- ☐ ....
- ☐ ....
- ☐ ....
- ☐ ....
- ☐ ....
- ☐ ....
- ☐ ....
- ☐ ....
- ☐ ....

TUESDAY — October 5

- ☐ ....
- ☐ ....
- ☐ ....
- ☐ ....
- ☐ ....
- ☐ ....
- ☐ ....
- ☐ ....
- ☐ ....
- ☐ ....
- ☐ ....
- ☐ ....
- ☐ ....
- ☐ ....

WEDNESDAY — October 6

- ☐ ....
- ☐ ....
- ☐ ....
- ☐ ....
- ☐ ....
- ☐ ....
- ☐ ....
- ☐ ....
- ☐ ....
- ☐ ....
- ☐ ....
- ☐ ....
- ☐ ....
- ☐ ....

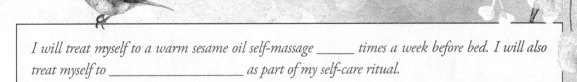

I will treat myself to a warm sesame oil self-massage _____ times a week before bed. I will also treat myself to _____ as part of my self-care ritual.

THURSDAY	FRIDAY	WEEKEND
October 7	October 8	October 9-10

☐ ....
☐ ....
☐ ....
☐ ....
☐ ....
☐ ....
☐ ....
☐ ....
☐ ....
☐ ....
☐ ....
☐ ....
☐ ....

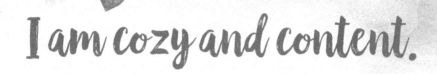

I am cozy and content.

MONDAY	TUESDAY	WEDNESDAY
October 11	October 12	October 13

MONDAY — October 11
- ☐ ....
- ☐ ....
- ☐ ....
- ☐ ....
- ☐ ....
- ☐ ....
- ☐ ....
- ☐ ....
- ☐ ....
- ☐ ....
- ☐ ....
- ☐ ....
- ☐ ....

TUESDAY — October 12
- ☐ ....
- ☐ ....
- ☐ ....
- ☐ ....
- ☐ ....
- ☐ ....
- ☐ ....
- ☐ ....
- ☐ ....
- ☐ ....
- ☐ ....
- ☐ ....
- ☐ ....

WEDNESDAY — October 13
- ☐ ....
- ☐ ....
- ☐ ....
- ☐ ....
- ☐ ....
- ☐ ....
- ☐ ....
- ☐ ....
- ☐ ....
- ☐ ....
- ☐ ....
- ☐ ....
- ☐ ....

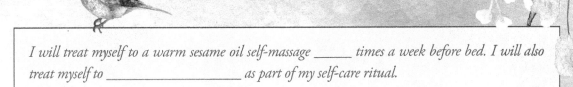

I will treat myself to a warm sesame oil self-massage _____ times a week before bed. I will also treat myself to _____ as part of my self-care ritual.

THURSDAY

October 14

- ☐ ....
- ☐ ....
- ☐ ....
- ☐ ....
- ☐ ....
- ☐ ....
- ☐ ....
- ☐ ....
- ☐ ....
- ☐ ....
- ☐ ....
- ☐ ....
- ☐ ....

FRIDAY

October 15

- ☐ ....
- ☐ ....
- ☐ ....
- ☐ ....
- ☐ ....
- ☐ ....
- ☐ ....
- ☐ ....
- ☐ ....
- ☐ ....
- ☐ ....
- ☐ ....
- ☐ ....

WEEKEND

October 16-17

- ☐ ....
- ☐ ....
- ☐ ....
- ☐ ....
- ☐ ....
- ☐ ....
- ☐ ....
- ☐ ....
- ☐ ....
- ☐ ....
- ☐ ....
- ☐ ....
- ☐ ....

I am enough.

MONDAY	TUESDAY	WEDNESDAY
October 18	October 19	October 20

MONDAY — October 18

- [ ] ....
- [ ] ....
- [ ] ....
- [ ] ....
- [ ] ....
- [ ] ....
- [ ] ....
- [ ] ....
- [ ] ....
- [ ] ....
- [ ] ....
- [ ] ....
- [ ] ....
- [ ] ....

TUESDAY — October 19

- [ ] ....
- [ ] ....
- [ ] ....
- [ ] ....
- [ ] ....
- [ ] ....
- [ ] ....
- [ ] ....
- [ ] ....
- [ ] ....
- [ ] ....
- [ ] ....
- [ ] ....
- [ ] ....

WEDNESDAY — October 20

- [ ] ....
- [ ] ....
- [ ] ....
- [ ] ....
- [ ] ....
- [ ] ....
- [ ] ....
- [ ] ....
- [ ] ....
- [ ] ....
- [ ] ....
- [ ] ....
- [ ] ....
- [ ] ....

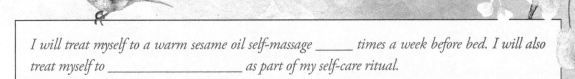

I will treat myself to a warm sesame oil self-massage _____ times a week before bed. I will also treat myself to _____ as part of my self-care ritual.

THURSDAY

October 21

- [ ] ....
- [ ] ....
- [ ] ....
- [ ] ....
- [ ] ....
- [ ] ....
- [ ] ....
- [ ] ....
- [ ] ....
- [ ] ....
- [ ] ....
- [ ] ....

FRIDAY

October 22

- [ ] ....
- [ ] ....
- [ ] ....
- [ ] ....
- [ ] ....
- [ ] ....
- [ ] ....
- [ ] ....
- [ ] ....
- [ ] ....
- [ ] ....
- [ ] ....

WEEKEND

October 23-24

- [ ] ....
- [ ] ....
- [ ] ....
- [ ] ....
- [ ] ....
- [ ] ....
- [ ] ....
- [ ] ....
- [ ] ....
- [ ] ....
- [ ] ....
- [ ] ....

I am encouraged.

MONDAY	TUESDAY	WEDNESDAY
October 25	October 26	October 27

- ☐ ....
- ☐ ....
- ☐ ....
- ☐ ....
- ☐ ....
- ☐ ....
- ☐ ....
- ☐ ....
- ☐ ....
- ☐ ....
- ☐ ....
- ☐ ....
- ☐ ....
- ☐ ....

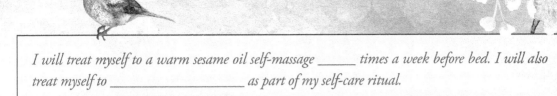

I will treat myself to a warm sesame oil self-massage _____ times a week before bed. I will also treat myself to _____ as part of my self-care ritual.

THURSDAY

October 28

- [ ] ....
- [ ] ....
- [ ] ....
- [ ] ....
- [ ] ....
- [ ] ....
- [ ] ....
- [ ] ....
- [ ] ....
- [ ] ....
- [ ] ....
- [ ] ....
- [ ] ....
- [ ] ....

FRIDAY

October 29

- [ ] ....
- [ ] ....
- [ ] ....
- [ ] ....
- [ ] ....
- [ ] ....
- [ ] ....
- [ ] ....
- [ ] ....
- [ ] ....
- [ ] ....
- [ ] ....
- [ ] ....
- [ ] ....

WEEKEND

October 30-31

- [ ] ....
- [ ] ....
- [ ] ....
- [ ] ....
- [ ] ....
- [ ] ....
- [ ] ....
- [ ] ....
- [ ] ....
- [ ] ....
- [ ] ....
- [ ] ....
- [ ] ....

STUFFED EGGPLANT

INGREDIENTS

- 1 MEDIUM EGGPLANT
- 1/2 CUP CHOPPED ONION
- 2 GARLIC CLOVES, MINCED
- 1/2 CUP CHOPPED FRESH MUSHROOMS
- 1/2 CUP CHOPPED ZUCCHINI
- 1/2 CUP CHOPPED SWEET RED PEPPER
- 3/4 CUP SEEDED CHOPPED TOMATOES
- 1/4 CUP TOASTED WHEAT GERM
- 2 TABLESPOONS MINCED FRESH PARSLEY
- 1/2 TEASPOON DRIED THYME
- 1/4 TEASPOON SALT
- 1/4 TEASPOON PEPPER
- DASH CRUSHED RED PEPPER FLAKES
- 1 TABLESPOON GRATED PARMESAN CHEESE

DIRECTIONS

Cut eggplant in half lengthwise; remove pulp, leaving a 1/4-in.-thick shell. Cube pulp; set shells and pulp aside. In a large nonstick skillet coated with cooking spray, sauté onion and garlic until onion is ten-der. Add the mushrooms, zucchini, red pepper and eggplant pulp; sauté for 4-6 minutes or un-til vegetables are crisp-tender. Stir in the tomatoes, wheat germ, parsley, thyme, salt, pepper and pepper flakes; cook for 1 minute. Divide mixture evenly between the eggplant shells; sprinkle with Parmesan cheese. Place on a baking sheet. Bake at 400° for 20-25 minutes or until shells are tender.

OJAS MILK

INGREDIENTS

- 1 CUP OF ALMOND MILK
- 1 TEASPOON OF GOLDEN MILK POWDER (WELLBLENDS)
- 3 DATES
- 1 PINCH OF SAFFRON

DIRECTIONS: Combine ingredients in a blender and blend. Serve room temperature or warm.

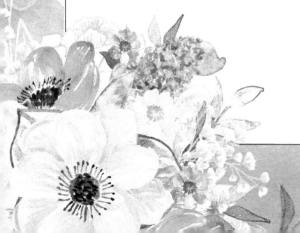

Journal

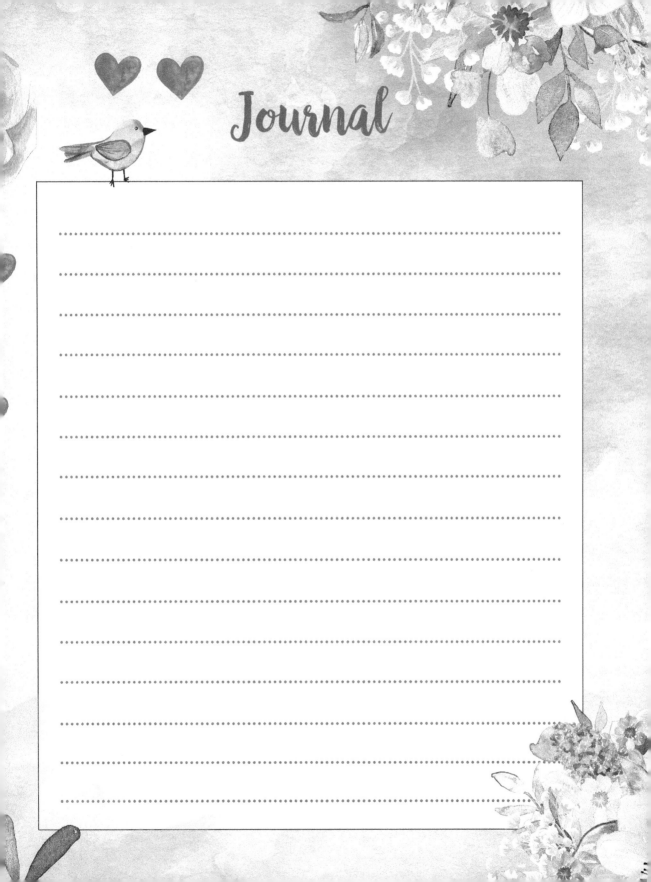

November

TO DO:

- ●
- ●
- ●
- ●
- ●
- ●
- ●
- ●
- ●
- ●
- ●
- ●

SUNDAY	MONDAY	TUESDAY
	1	2
7 *Nourish*	8	9
14	15	16
21	22	23 *Moisturize*
28	29	30

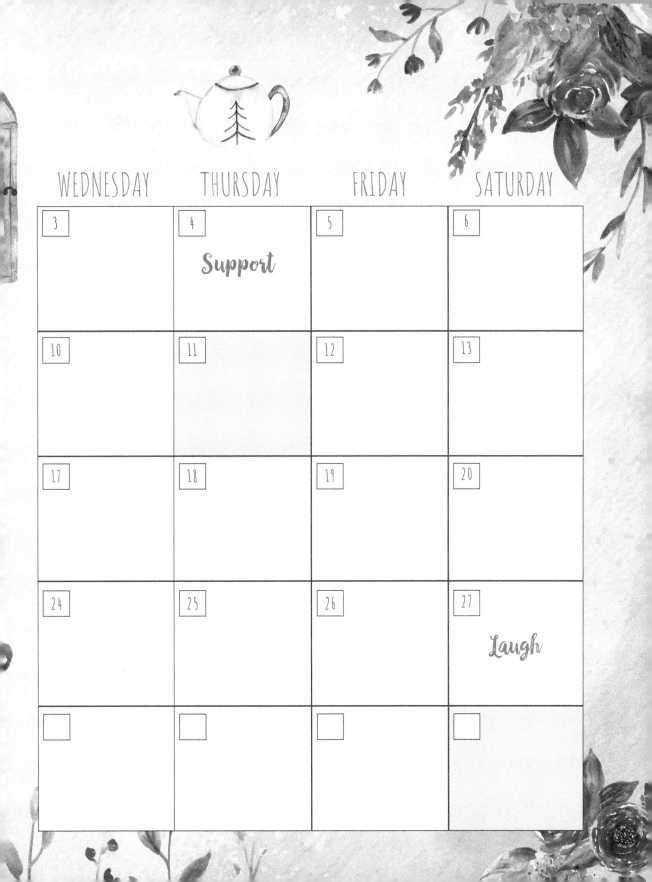

WEDNESDAY	THURSDAY	FRIDAY	SATURDAY
3	4 *Support*	5	6
10	11	12	13
17	18	19	20
24	25	26	27 *Laugh*
☐	☐	☐	☐

I am grateful.

MONDAY

November 1

- ☐ ....
- ☐ ....
- ☐ ....
- ☐ ....
- ☐ ....
- ☐ ....
- ☐ ....
- ☐ ....
- ☐ ....
- ☐ ....
- ☐ ....
- ☐ ....
- ☐ ....

TUESDAY

November 2

- ☐ ....
- ☐ ....
- ☐ ....
- ☐ ....
- ☐ ....
- ☐ ....
- ☐ ....
- ☐ ....
- ☐ ....
- ☐ ....
- ☐ ....
- ☐ ....
- ☐ ....

WEDNESDAY

November 3

- ☐ ....
- ☐ ....
- ☐ ....
- ☐ ....
- ☐ ....
- ☐ ....
- ☐ ....
- ☐ ....
- ☐ ....
- ☐ ....
- ☐ ....
- ☐ ....
- ☐ ....

I nourish myself with warm foods for lunch and soothe myself with golden milk at night. This week I will make _____. (soup, stir-fry, spiced porridge, ect)

THURSDAY

November 4

- [ ] ....
- [ ] ....
- [ ] ....
- [ ] ....
- [ ] ....
- [ ] ....
- [ ] ....
- [ ] ....
- [ ] ....
- [ ] ....
- [ ] ....
- [ ] ....
- [ ] ....
- [ ] ....

FRIDAY

November 5

- [ ] ....
- [ ] ....
- [ ] ....
- [ ] ....
- [ ] ....
- [ ] ....
- [ ] ....
- [ ] ....
- [ ] ....
- [ ] ....
- [ ] ....
- [ ] ....
- [ ] ....
- [ ] ....

WEEKEND

November 6-7

- [ ] ....
- [ ] ....
- [ ] ....
- [ ] ....
- [ ] ....
- [ ] ....
- [ ] ....
- [ ] ....
- [ ] ....
- [ ] ....
- [ ] ....
- [ ] ....
- [ ] ....
- [ ] ....

I am present.

MONDAY	TUESDAY	WEDNESDAY
November 8	November 9	November 10

MONDAY — November 8

- ☐ ....
- ☐ ....
- ☐ ....
- ☐ ....
- ☐ ....
- ☐ ....
- ☐ ....
- ☐ ....
- ☐ ....
- ☐ ....
- ☐ ....
- ☐ ....
- ☐ ....

TUESDAY — November 9

- ☐ ....
- ☐ ....
- ☐ ....
- ☐ ....
- ☐ ....
- ☐ ....
- ☐ ....
- ☐ ....
- ☐ ....
- ☐ ....
- ☐ ....
- ☐ ....
- ☐ ....

WEDNESDAY — November 10

- ☐ ....
- ☐ ....
- ☐ ....
- ☐ ....
- ☐ ....
- ☐ ....
- ☐ ....
- ☐ ....
- ☐ ....
- ☐ ....
- ☐ ....
- ☐ ....
- ☐ ....

I nourish myself with warm foods for lunch and soothe myself with golden milk at night. This week I will make _____. (soup, stir-fry, spiced porridge, ect)

THURSDAY

November 11

- [ ] ....
- [ ] ....
- [ ] ....
- [ ] ....
- [ ] ....
- [ ] ....
- [ ] ....
- [ ] ....
- [ ] ....
- [ ] ....
- [ ] ....
- [ ] ....
- [ ] ....

FRIDAY

November 12

- [ ] ....
- [ ] ....
- [ ] ....
- [ ] ....
- [ ] ....
- [ ] ....
- [ ] ....
- [ ] ....
- [ ] ....
- [ ] ....
- [ ] ....
- [ ] ....
- [ ] ....

WEEKEND

November 13-14

- [ ] ....
- [ ] ....
- [ ] ....
- [ ] ....
- [ ] ....
- [ ] ....
- [ ] ....
- [ ] ....
- [ ] ....
- [ ] ....
- [ ] ....
- [ ] ....
- [ ] ....

I am at ease.

MONDAY
November 15

- [ ] ....
- [ ] ....
- [ ] ....
- [ ] ....
- [ ] ....
- [ ] ....
- [ ] ....
- [ ] ....
- [ ] ....
- [ ] ....
- [ ] ....
- [ ] ....
- [ ] ....
- [ ] ....

TUESDAY
November 16

- [ ] ....
- [ ] ....
- [ ] ....
- [ ] ....
- [ ] ....
- [ ] ....
- [ ] ....
- [ ] ....
- [ ] ....
- [ ] ....
- [ ] ....
- [ ] ....
- [ ] ....
- [ ] ....

WEDNESDAY
November 17

- [ ] ....
- [ ] ....
- [ ] ....
- [ ] ....
- [ ] ....
- [ ] ....
- [ ] ....
- [ ] ....
- [ ] ....
- [ ] ....
- [ ] ....
- [ ] ....
- [ ] ....
- [ ] ....

I nourish myself with warm foods for lunch and soothe myself with golden milk at night. This week I will make _____. (soup, stir-fry, spiced porridge, ect)

THURSDAY
November 18

- [ ] ....
- [ ] ....
- [ ] ....
- [ ] ....
- [ ] ....
- [ ] ....
- [ ] ....
- [ ] ....
- [ ] ....
- [ ] ....
- [ ] ....
- [ ] ....
- [ ] ....

FRIDAY
November 19

- [ ] ....
- [ ] ....
- [ ] ....
- [ ] ....
- [ ] ....
- [ ] ....
- [ ] ....
- [ ] ....
- [ ] ....
- [ ] ....
- [ ] ....
- [ ] ....
- [ ] ....

WEEKEND
November 20-21

- [ ] ....
- [ ] ....
- [ ] ....
- [ ] ....
- [ ] ....
- [ ] ....
- [ ] ....
- [ ] ....
- [ ] ....
- [ ] ....
- [ ] ....
- [ ] ....
- [ ] ....

I am radiating positive energy.

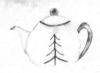

MONDAY	TUESDAY	WEDNESDAY
November 22	November 23	November 24

MONDAY — November 22

- ☐ ....
- ☐ ....
- ☐ ....
- ☐ ....
- ☐ ....
- ☐ ....
- ☐ ....
- ☐ ....
- ☐ ....
- ☐ ....
- ☐ ....
- ☐ ....
- ☐ ....
- ☐ ....

TUESDAY — November 23

- ☐ ....
- ☐ ....
- ☐ ....
- ☐ ....
- ☐ ....
- ☐ ....
- ☐ ....
- ☐ ....
- ☐ ....
- ☐ ....
- ☐ ....
- ☐ ....
- ☐ ....
- ☐ ....

WEDNESDAY — November 24

- ☐ ....
- ☐ ....
- ☐ ....
- ☐ ....
- ☐ ....
- ☐ ....
- ☐ ....
- ☐ ....
- ☐ ....
- ☐ ....
- ☐ ....
- ☐ ....
- ☐ ....
- ☐ ....

I nourish myself with warm foods for lunch and soothe myself with golden milk at night. This week I will make _____. (soup, stir-fry, spiced porridge, ect)

THURSDAY

November 25

- ☐ ....
- ☐ ....
- ☐ ....
- ☐ ....
- ☐ ....
- ☐ ....
- ☐ ....
- ☐ ....
- ☐ ....
- ☐ ....
- ☐ ....
- ☐ ....
- ☐ ....

FRIDAY

November 26

- ☐ ....
- ☐ ....
- ☐ ....
- ☐ ....
- ☐ ....
- ☐ ....
- ☐ ....
- ☐ ....
- ☐ ....
- ☐ ....
- ☐ ....
- ☐ ....
- ☐ ....

WEEKEND

November 27-28

- ☐ ....
- ☐ ....
- ☐ ....
- ☐ ....
- ☐ ....
- ☐ ....
- ☐ ....
- ☐ ....
- ☐ ....
- ☐ ....
- ☐ ....
- ☐ ....

I am centered.

MONDAY	TUESDAY	WEDNESDAY
November 29	November 30	December 1

Journal

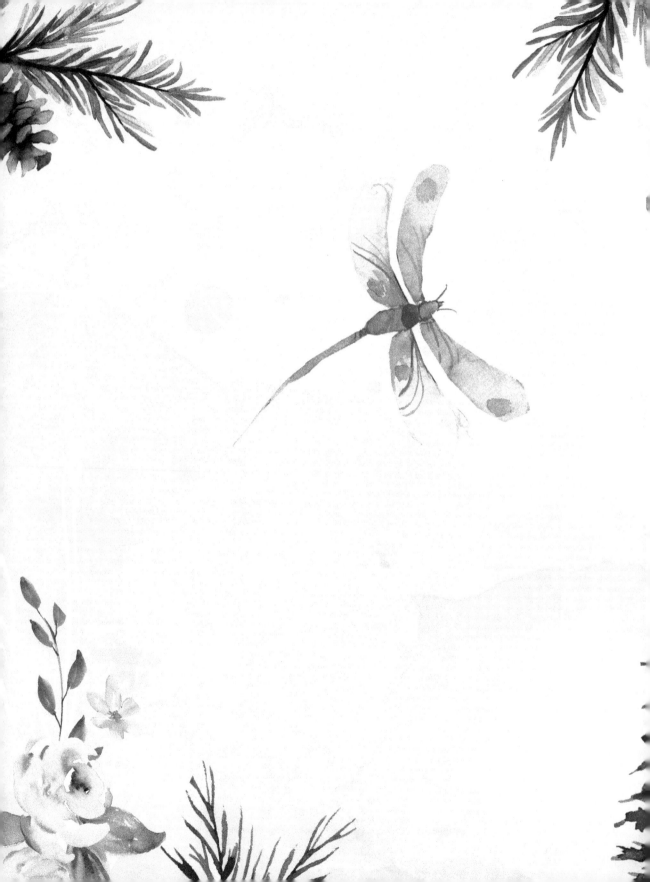

BEST TEAS

for the Holiday Season:

- GINGER TEA AND PEPPERMINT FOR DIGESTION (DETOX & REPLENISH BY WELLBLENDS)

- CHAMAMILE TEA AND GOLDEN MILK FOR RELAXATION.

- ECHINACEA TEA AND GREEN TEA FOR IMMUNITY.

ESSENTIAL OILS

Tool Kit:

- THIEVES OIL AND OREGANO OIL FOR IMMUNITY

- LAVENDER AND YLANG YLANG FOR RELAXATION

- SPEARMINT AND SWEET ORANGE ESSENTIAL OILS FOR ENERGY

December

TO DO:

SUNDAY

MONDAY

TUESDAY

SUNDAY	MONDAY	TUESDAY
☐	☐	☐
5	6	7
12	13 *Joy*	14
19	20	21
26 *Self-care*	27	28

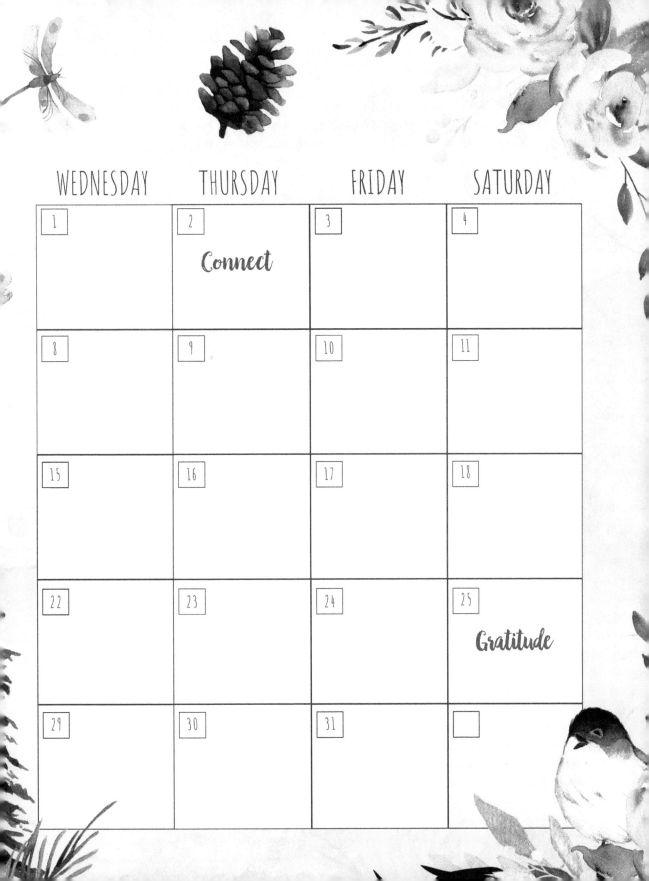

WEDNESDAY	THURSDAY	FRIDAY	SATURDAY
1	2 Connect	3	4
8	9	10	11
15	16	17	18
22	23	24	25 Gratitude
29	30	31	

I am abundant.

MONDAY	TUESDAY	WEDNESDAY
November 29	November 30	December 1

MONDAY — November 29

- ☐ ....
- ☐ ....
- ☐ ....
- ☐ ....
- ☐ ....
- ☐ ....
- ☐ ....
- ☐ ....
- ☐ ....
- ☐ ....
- ☐ ....
- ☐ ....
- ☐ ....
- ☐ ....

TUESDAY — November 30

- ☐ ....
- ☐ ....
- ☐ ....
- ☐ ....
- ☐ ....
- ☐ ....
- ☐ ....
- ☐ ....
- ☐ ....
- ☐ ....
- ☐ ....
- ☐ ....
- ☐ ....
- ☐ ....

WEDNESDAY — December 1

- ☐ ....
- ☐ ....
- ☐ ....
- ☐ ....
- ☐ ....
- ☐ ....
- ☐ ....
- ☐ ....
- ☐ ....
- ☐ ....
- ☐ ....
- ☐ ....
- ☐ ....
- ☐ ....

Weekly Aims: I am committed to the staples that bring me balance:

My teas this week _____.

My essential oils this week _____.

My movement this week _____.

THURSDAY

December 2

- [ ] ....
- [ ] ....
- [ ] ....
- [ ] ....
- [ ] ....
- [ ] ....
- [ ] ....
- [ ] ....
- [ ] ....
- [ ] ....
- [ ] ....
- [ ] ....
- [ ] ....

FRIDAY

December 3

- [ ] ....
- [ ] ....
- [ ] ....
- [ ] ....
- [ ] ....
- [ ] ....
- [ ] ....
- [ ] ....
- [ ] ....
- [ ] ....
- [ ] ....
- [ ] ....
- [ ] ....

WEEKEND

December 4-5

- [ ] ....
- [ ] ....
- [ ] ....
- [ ] ....
- [ ] ....
- [ ] ....
- [ ] ....
- [ ] ....
- [ ] ....
- [ ] ....
- [ ] ....
- [ ] ....
- [ ] ....

I am allowed to say no.

MONDAY	TUESDAY	WEDNESDAY
December 6	December 7	December 8

MONDAY — December 6

- ☐ ....
- ☐ ....
- ☐ ....
- ☐ ....
- ☐ ....
- ☐ ....
- ☐ ....
- ☐ ....
- ☐ ....
- ☐ ....
- ☐ ....
- ☐ ....
- ☐ ....

TUESDAY — December 7

- ☐ ....
- ☐ ....
- ☐ ....
- ☐ ....
- ☐ ....
- ☐ ....
- ☐ ....
- ☐ ....
- ☐ ....
- ☐ ....
- ☐ ....
- ☐ ....
- ☐ ....

WEDNESDAY — December 8

- ☐ ....
- ☐ ....
- ☐ ....
- ☐ ....
- ☐ ....
- ☐ ....
- ☐ ....
- ☐ ....
- ☐ ....
- ☐ ....
- ☐ ....
- ☐ ....
- ☐ ....

Weekly Aims: I am committed to the staples that bring me balance:
My teas this week _____.
My essential oils this week _____.
My movement this week _____.

THURSDAY

December 9

- [ ] ....
- [ ] ....
- [ ] ....
- [ ] ....
- [ ] ....
- [ ] ....
- [ ] ....
- [ ] ....
- [ ] ....
- [ ] ....
- [ ] ....
- [ ] ....
- [ ] ....
- [ ] ....

FRIDAY

December 10

- [ ] ....
- [ ] ....
- [ ] ....
- [ ] ....
- [ ] ....
- [ ] ....
- [ ] ....
- [ ] ....
- [ ] ....
- [ ] ....
- [ ] ....
- [ ] ....
- [ ] ....
- [ ] ....

WEEKEND

December 11-12

- [ ] ....
- [ ] ....
- [ ] ....
- [ ] ....
- [ ] ....
- [ ] ....
- [ ] ....
- [ ] ....
- [ ] ....
- [ ] ....
- [ ] ....
- [ ] ....
- [ ] ....

I am of joyful.

MONDAY
December 13

- [ ] ....
- [ ] ....
- [ ] ....
- [ ] ....
- [ ] ....
- [ ] ....
- [ ] ....
- [ ] ....
- [ ] ....
- [ ] ....
- [ ] ....
- [ ] ....
- [ ] ....

TUESDAY
December 14

- [ ] ....
- [ ] ....
- [ ] ....
- [ ] ....
- [ ] ....
- [ ] ....
- [ ] ....
- [ ] ....
- [ ] ....
- [ ] ....
- [ ] ....
- [ ] ....
- [ ] ....

WEDNESDAY
December 15

- [ ] ....
- [ ] ....
- [ ] ....
- [ ] ....
- [ ] ....
- [ ] ....
- [ ] ....
- [ ] ....
- [ ] ....
- [ ] ....
- [ ] ....
- [ ] ....
- [ ] ....

Weekly Aims: I am committed to the staples that bring me balance:

My teas this week _____.

My essential oils this week _____.

My movement this week _____.

THURSDAY

December 16

- [ ] ....
- [ ] ....
- [ ] ....
- [ ] ....
- [ ] ....
- [ ] ....
- [ ] ....
- [ ] ....
- [ ] ....
- [ ] ....
- [ ] ....
- [ ] ....
- [ ] ....
- [ ] ....

FRIDAY

December 17

- [ ] ....
- [ ] ....
- [ ] ....
- [ ] ....
- [ ] ....
- [ ] ....
- [ ] ....
- [ ] ....
- [ ] ....
- [ ] ....
- [ ] ....
- [ ] ....
- [ ] ....
- [ ] ....

WEEKEND

December 18-19

- [ ] ....
- [ ] ....
- [ ] ....
- [ ] ....
- [ ] ....
- [ ] ....
- [ ] ....
- [ ] ....
- [ ] ....
- [ ] ....
- [ ] ....
- [ ] ....
- [ ] ....
- [ ] ....

I am making choices that align with my intentions.

MONDAY	TUESDAY	WEDNESDAY
December 20	December 21	December 22

MONDAY — December 20
- ☐ ....
- ☐ ....
- ☐ ....
- ☐ ....
- ☐ ....
- ☐ ....
- ☐ ....
- ☐ ....
- ☐ ....
- ☐ ....
- ☐ ....
- ☐ ....
- ☐ ....

TUESDAY — December 21
- ☐ ....
- ☐ ....
- ☐ ....
- ☐ ....
- ☐ ....
- ☐ ....
- ☐ ....
- ☐ ....
- ☐ ....
- ☐ ....
- ☐ ....
- ☐ ....
- ☐ ....

WEDNESDAY — December 22
- ☐ ....
- ☐ ....
- ☐ ....
- ☐ ....
- ☐ ....
- ☐ ....
- ☐ ....
- ☐ ....
- ☐ ....
- ☐ ....
- ☐ ....
- ☐ ....
- ☐ ....

Weekly Aims: I am committed to the staples that bring me balance:

My teas this week _____.

My essential oils this week _____.

My movement this week _____.

THURSDAY
December 23

☐ ....
☐ ....
☐ ....
☐ ....
☐ ....
☐ ....
☐ ....
☐ ....
☐ ....
☐ ....
☐ ....
☐ ....
☐ ....

FRIDAY
December 24

☐ ....
☐ ....
☐ ....
☐ ....
☐ ....
☐ ....
☐ ....
☐ ....
☐ ....
☐ ....
☐ ....
☐ ....
☐ ....

WEEKEND
December 25-26

☐ ....
☐ ....
☐ ....
☐ ....
☐ ....
☐ ....
☐ ....
☐ ....
☐ ....
☐ ....
☐ ....
☐ ....
☐ ....

I am content.

MONDAY	TUESDAY	WEDNESDAY
December 27	December 28	December 29

MONDAY — December 27

- ☐ ....
- ☐ ....
- ☐ ....
- ☐ ....
- ☐ ....
- ☐ ....
- ☐ ....
- ☐ ....
- ☐ ....
- ☐ ....
- ☐ ....
- ☐ ....
- ☐ ....

TUESDAY — December 28

- ☐ ....
- ☐ ....
- ☐ ....
- ☐ ....
- ☐ ....
- ☐ ....
- ☐ ....
- ☐ ....
- ☐ ....
- ☐ ....
- ☐ ....
- ☐ ....
- ☐ ....

WEDNESDAY — December 29

- ☐ ....
- ☐ ....
- ☐ ....
- ☐ ....
- ☐ ....
- ☐ ....
- ☐ ....
- ☐ ....
- ☐ ....
- ☐ ....
- ☐ ....
- ☐ ....
- ☐ ....

Weekly Aims: *I am committed to the staples that bring me balance:*
My teas this week _____.
My essential oils this week _____.
My movement this week _____.

THURSDAY	FRIDAY	WEEKEND
December 30	December 31	January 1-2
☐	☐	☐ ....
☐	☐	☐ ....
☐	☐	☐ ....
☐	☐	☐ ....
☐	☐	☐ ....
☐	☐	☐ ....
☐	☐	☐ ....
☐	☐	☐ ....
☐	☐	☐ ....
☐	☐	☐ ....
☐	☐	☐ ....
☐	☐	☐ ....
☐	☐	☐ ....

Journal

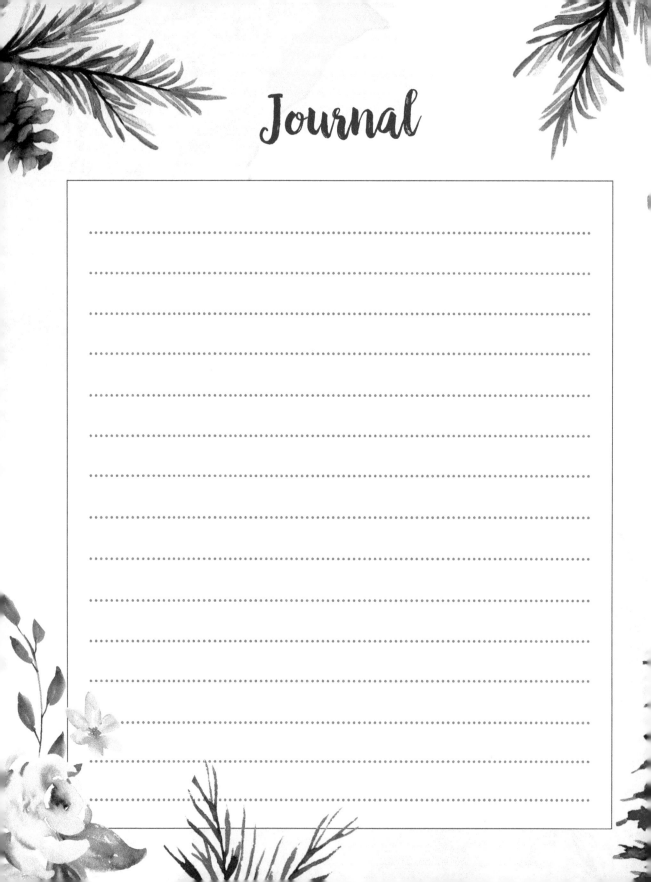

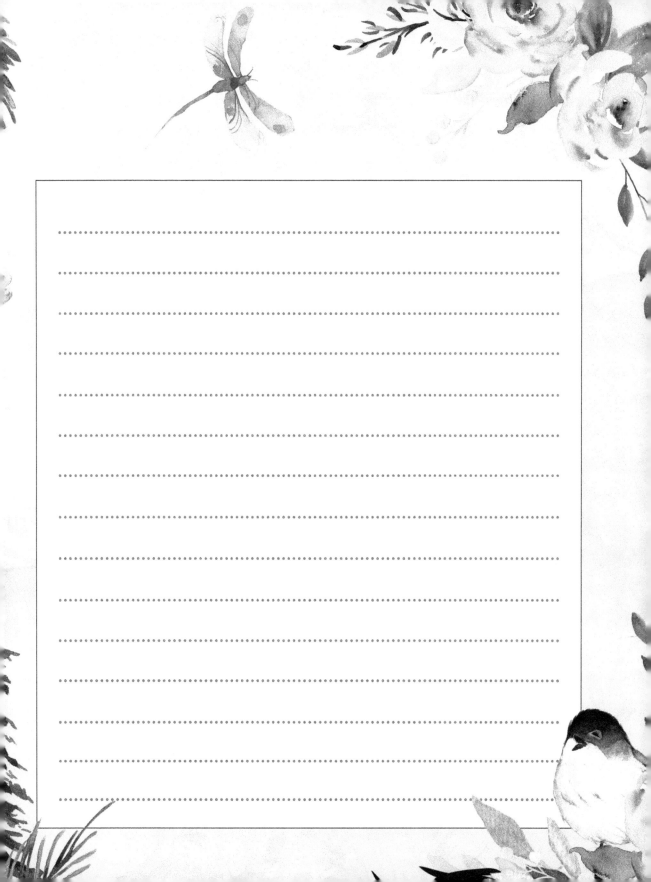

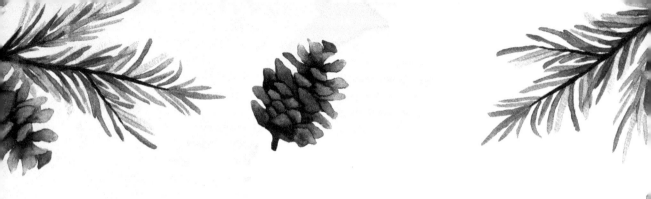

Organic Ayurvedic Products for Self-Care:

teas, golden milk and more

WWW.WELLBLENDS.COM

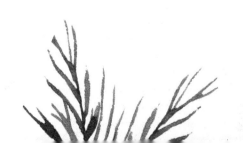

CPSIA information can be obtained
at www.ICGtesting.com
Printed in the USA
LVHW022237120121
676264LV00009BA/176